*Perspectives in
Nursing 1991–1993*

Perspectives in Nursing 1991–1993

National League for Nursing Press • New York
Pub. No. 41-2472

Copyright © 1992
National League for Nursing
350 Hudson Street, New York, NY 10014

All rights reserved. No part of this book may be reproduced in print, or by photostatic means, or in any other manner, without the express written permission of the publisher.

ISBN 0-88737-550-2

> The views expressed in this publication represent the views of the authors and do not necessarily reflect the official views of the National League for Nursing.

This book was set in Palatino by Publications Development Company of Texas. The editor was Janice Weisner; the designer was Andrea Arvonio. Northeastern Press was the printer and binder.

The cover was designed by Lillian Welsh.

Printed in the United States of America

Contents

CONTRIBUTORS	ix
PREFACE	xi

Nursing's Agenda for the 21st Century — 1

1 NURSING AND SOCIETY—THE UNFINISHED AGENDA FOR THE 21ST CENTURY — 3
Donna E. Shalala

Trends in Nursing Education — 9

2 RECENT TRENDS IN NURSING EDUCATION — 11
Peri Rosenfeld

Cultural Diversity in Nursing Education — 21

3 QUALITY EDUCATION FOR MINORITIES: MYTHS, REALITIES, AND STRATEGIES — 23
Shirley M. McBay

4 DIVERSITY IN NURSING FACULTY HINGES ON DIVERSITY IN NURSING STUDENTS — 35
Sallie Tucker-Allen

v

5	EDUCATIONAL IMPLICATIONS OF NURSING FACULTY DIVERSITY	43
	Ruby L. Steele	
6	VALUING CULTURAL DIVERSITY IN NURSING FACULTY	47
	Joanette Pete McGadney	
7	NURSING FROM THE INTERNATIONAL PERSPECTIVE	53
	Jeanette Lancaster	

Nursing and the Community   59

8	A COMMUNITY-BASED HEALTH PROGRAM FOR THE HOMELESS	61
	Tim Porter-O'Grady and Lorine Spencer	
9	NURSING AND COMMUNITY ADVOCACY: HEALTH NEEDS OF THE YOUNG	71
	Jeannette O. Poindexter	
10	A CHURCH-BASED PROGRAM FOR THE HOMELESS	77
	Cora Newell-Withrow	
11	PREVENTION AS THE INTERVENTION OF CHOICE	83
	Mae E. Markstrom and Kathryn Fiandt	

Distance Education and New Technology   93

12	DISTANCE EDUCATION: TURF AND TECHNOLOGY	95
	Myrna R. Pickard	
13	DISTANT LEARNING IN NURSING	99
	Michael A. Carter	
14	DISTANCE EDUCATION: TURF AND TECHNOLOGY	105
	Thelma Cleveland	

Contents vii

Alternative Nursing Practice 111

15 CASE MANAGEMENT: WITHIN AND BEYOND
    THE WALLS 113
    Helen R. Connors

16 A CARING COMMUNITY WITHIN ACUTE-CARE
    INSTITUTIONS? IT CAN BE DONE, AND HERE'S HOW 121
    Eloise M. Balasco

17 VIOLENCE AGAINST WOMEN: CLINICAL ISSUES 127
    Josephine Ryan and Christine King

Legal and Economic Challenges for the Decade 135

18 HOME CARE: THE DIRECTION OF FUTURE
    HEALTH CARE SERVICES 137
    Cathy Frasca

19 COMPETITION IN ACCREDITING: LETTING
    OTHER VOICES BE HEARD 147
    Clark C. Havighurst

Reevaluating Nursing's Agenda 159

20 PRESIDENTIAL ADDRESS FOR THE BIENNIAL
    CONVENTION 161
    Patty Hawken

21 COMMUNITY-BASED NURSING EDUCATION IN
    EL SALVADOR 167
    Rosa Rodriguez-Deras

22 HERE THERE BE DRAGONS: DEPARTING THE
    BEHAVIORIST PARADIGM FOR STATE BOARD
    REGULATION 177
    Julia E. Gould and Em Olivia Bevis

Contributors

Eloise M. Balasco, MSN, RN, is Vice President, Nursing, Mercy Hospital, Portland, Maine.

Em Olivia Bevis, EdD, RN, FAAN, is Consultant in Nursing Education and Adjunct Professor, Research, Georgia Southern University, Statesboro, Georgia.

Michael A. Carter, DNSc, RN, FAAN, is Dean, College of Nursing, University of Tennessee, Memphis, Tennessee.

Thelma Cleveland, PhD, RN, is Dean, Intercollegiate Center for Nursing Education, Spokane, Washington.

Helen R. Connors, PhD, RN, is Assistant Professor, School of Nursing, University of Kansas, Kansas City, Kansas.

Kathryn Fiandt, MSN, FNP, RN, C, is Clinical Director, Wellness Care Center, Lake Superior State University, Saulte Sainte Marie, Michigan.

Cathy Frasca, BSN, RN FACHA, is Executive Director, South Hills Health System Home Health Agency, Homestead, Pennsylvania.

Julia E. Gould, MS, RN, is Nursing Education Consultant, Georgia Board of Nursing, Atlanta, Georgia.

Clark C. Havighurst, JD, AB, is William Neal Reynolds Professor of Law, School of Law, Duke University, Durham, North Carolina.

Patty Hawken, PhD, RN, FAAN, is President, National League for Nursing, New York, New York.

Christine King, EdD, RN, is Assistant Professor, School of Nursing, University of Massachusetts, Amherst, Massachusetts.

Jeanette Lancaster, PhD, RN, FAAN, is Sadie Heath Cabiniss Professor and Dean, School of Nursing, University of Virginia, Charlottesville, Virginia.

Mae E. Markstrom, PhD, RN, is Head, Department of Health Sciences, Lake Superior State University, Saulte Sainte Marie, Michigan.

Shirley M. McBay, PhD, is President, Quality Education for Minorities Network, Washington, DC.

Joanette Pete McGadney, PhD, RN, is Associate Professor and Chairperson, Department of Nursing, University of West Florida.

Cora Newell-Withrow, DSN, RN, FAAN, is Professor and Chair, Department of Nursing, Berea College, Berea, Kentucky.

Myrna R. Pickard, EdD, RN, is Professor and Dean, School of Nursing, University of Texas, Arlington, Texas.

Jeannette O. Poindexter, PhD, FAAN, is Associate Professor, College of Nursing, Wayne State University, Detroit, Michigan.

Tim Porter-O'Grady, EdD, RN, CS, CNAA, FAAN, is Senior Partner of TPOG, Inc., Atlanta, Georgia.

Rosa Rodriguez-Deras, MA, RN, is Dean, School of Medical Technology, National University of El Salvador, San Salvador, El Salvador.

Peri Rosenfeld, PhD, is Vice President, Division of Research, National League for Nursing, New York, New York.

Josephine Ryan, DNSc, RN, is Assistant Professor, School of Nursing, University of Amherst, Amherst, Massachusetts.

Donna E. Shalala, PhD, is Chancellor, University of Wisconsin, Madison, Wisconsin.

Lorine Spencer, MBA, RN, is Executive Director, Atlanta Community Health Program, Atlanta, Georgia.

Ruby L. Steele, PhD, RN, is Associate Professor, Department of Nursing, Southwest Missouri State University, Cape Girardeau, Missouri.

Sallie Tucker-Allen, PhD, RN, FAAN, is Associate Professor and Chair, Department of Nursing, University of Wisconsin, Green Bay, Wisconsin.

Preface

*T*he National League for Nursing's biennial conventions are noted for the wealth of talent and expertise gathered in pursuit of enhanced understandings of current health care issues of national and international concern. The 1991 convention, held in Nashville, Tennessee, explored a theme that, in this political year, has assumed even greater significance: "Toward a Healthier Nation: Educating for Reality." This latest volume in the *PERSPECTIVES IN NURSING* series documents outstanding presentations from that convention as they were given and with only minor editorial changes.

Each of the papers included here emphasizes a particular position or focus on professional nursing and health care issues within the larger context of immediate cultural, social, and political needs as we move through the last decade of the 20th century.

The papers in this collection have been organized into eight parts to delineate areas of major concern. The first part, "Nursing's Agenda for the 21st Century," offers the convention keynote address which, moving from the gains fought for and won in previous decades, looks ahead to nursing's *unfinished agenda* for the 21st century. The second part, "Trends in Nursing Education," focuses on recent developments in demographic research and other data collection, areas in which NLN is an acknowledged leader. The third part, "Cultural Diversity in Nursing Education," broaches pertinent questions concerning education for minorities, implications of diversity in faculty, and the international perspective. The fourth part, "Nursing and the Community," expands upon the current debate on strategies of nursing advocacy for the homeless, the young, and the rural elderly. The fifth part, "Distance Education and New Technology," discusses possibilities of nursing education in rural settings as a measure of our ability to find appropriate pedagogical models for widely scattered student populations.

The sixth part, "Alternative Nursing Practice," promotes creative designs in case management for the independent frail elderly, sensitive caring within acute-care institutions, and clinical lessons to be gained from dealing with women who have suffered violence against themselves. The seventh part, "Legal and Economic Challenges for the Decade," examines such challenges within the burgeoning field of home care and to the burden of accreditation within the still largely held health care paradigm as defined by the *medical* establishment. Finally, the last part, "Reevaluating Nursing's Agenda," places the National League for Nursing at the forefront of national health care reform. In addition, this part offers two papers of special import: the transformation of health care and health care education in the brutalized country of El Salvador and, closer to home, a critique of behaviorist paradigms within state board regulations.

The issues raised in this volume come at a time when health care is a national and international priority. The controversies argued and strategies proposed enter the moment with full awareness of the need to maintain the highest standards of care with the most effective measures of intervention in health care issues. It is our hope that this volume will contribute something of the intelligence and compassion necessary to make the immediate future a healthier one.

Allan Graubard
Senior Editor
National League for Nursing

PART ONE

Nursing's Agenda for the 21st Century

1

Nursing and Society—The Unfinished Agenda for the 21st Century

Donna E. Shalala

I cannot think of a profession that has changed more in a generation than nursing. Nurse educators who are still active on our faculty at the University of Wisconsin remember the days when nurses were required to stand when a doctor walked into the room. The days of the nurse practitioner, the nursing researcher, the clinic owned and operated by nurses in private practice, the doctorate of nursing, once were far in the future. Nurses were the handmaids of the medical profession. And now, through the gallant and sometimes arduous efforts of women and men like yourselves, nursing has redefined itself. It has staked out its territory and that territory is health: Prevention, Self-sufficiency and mobility for the elderly, Care for the poor, Women's health, Health education. Any person who has had any contact with the health profession in the past ten years has experienced the strength and growth and revolution of the profession. Now nursing is increasingly a powerful political force, a compassionate force that seeks to address the gross inequities of the way health care is delivered in our country. Nurses, who were once the handmaids, who now are the shock troops, understand, more intimately than anyone, the problems of people trapped in our city's concrete canyons or stranded in rural pockets of poverty.

You, more than anyone, as President Hawken has stated so eloquently, grieve at the realization that the great advances of science are available mostly to the few, while the many go without even the basics every American has the right to expect: Immunization, well-baby care, prenatal care, good nutrition. You feel the alarm at the numbers.

Health care is expected to cost more than $756 billion dollars in 1991 alone. You know what those numbers mean. You share the fear and despair of uninsured working people, trying to protect their families. You see the anguish of families whose life savings are drained away by nursing home care.

Because of some of the important work of our own school of nursing at Wisconsin, I am familiar with the great efforts nursing has made on behalf of the elderly. Major work on the link between teaching and nursing homes has come out of our university, in connection with many others. Nurses have undergone more extensive educational preparation and taken expanded roles in nursing homes, working for autonomy, quality of care and restorative therapy. Nursing educators have helped students understand the professional and personal rewards of working with our oldest citizens. And, changes are being made that will make nursing homes really deserve their names. Places to restore health instead of way stations on the road to dying. Nursing educators, policy makers, and medical researchers have done an enormously successful job in recent years in assuring better quality of life for our elderly.

That is only just. That is a cause for celebration. There continues to be work to be done for our elderly, but we must also turn our attention increasingly to the little ones who have no voices, no political clout, no voters' registration. A few months ago, Edward Zigler, the renowned child-development specialist from Yale, said bluntly, "We have never seen the plight of American children as bad as it is today." Tom Downey, a congressman from New York, told a congressional subcommittee last month that we should be proud of what we have done for our elderly and horrified at what we're doing for our children.

My own involvement with the needs of our poorest children extends back many years and is, in a sense, selfish. The girl who could be president of the class of 2005 at UW is playing in a courtyard filled with broken bottles at the Robert Taylor Homes in Chicago. A future archaeologist might be living outside Memphis today, in a trailer with no running water. A future nurse practitioner is 16 months old and living in Milwaukee, where her teenage mother, pregnant again, is so overburdened and lost that she cannot even provide fresh milk and a clean place to sleep. The judges and teachers and scientists and engineers of the future are entering overcrowded school systems in Boston, where they will be brushed to the side by children with problems even more terrible than their own. The future scholar—teachers at this nation's finest schools and colleges of nursing are being introduced to drugs—or born as crack babies in New York and Los Angeles.

Years ago, I became involved with the Children's Defense Fund, which was founded by my friend, Marian Wright Edelman. Marian has said for decades that saving our poorest children is our best investment in *our own* futures. They will grow up beside our own children. These children may never contribute to Social Security. They may absorb much, much more than their share of health resources and, in turn, produce children who will need expensive health care all their lives. They will use public safety resources, school remedial programs. They will wreck homes instead of building them. These children may grow up to take and take and take and never once give back.

Though the media was recently able to rivet the compassion of Americans on the plight of suffering citizens in Kuwait, it has been a harder job enlisting our interest in preserving our own most precious resource. Today there is a great celebration ticker tape parade in New York City. There are more children at risk in a two-mile radius of that parade than ever were at risk in the Persian Gulf.

Let me share with you one day in the life of American children. In one day in the wealthiest nation on earth, two thousand, seven hundred and ninety-five teenagers get pregnant. One thousand, one hundred and six teenagers have abortions. One thousand, two hundred and ninety-five girls give birth. Seven hundred babies are born to mothers who have had little or no prenatal care. Seven hundred more are born low birthweight. Sixty-seven babies under one month of age die. One hundred and five babies die before their first birthday. Twenty-seven children die from no other cause than the effects of poverty. One day in the wealthiest nation on earth, three die from child abuse. Ten die from guns. Thirty are wounded by guns, but survive. One hundred and thirty-five thousand American children—*in one day*—bring guns to school. Six teens commit suicide. Four hundred and thirty-seven children are arrested for drunk driving. One thousand, five hundred children drop out of school. Two hundred and eleven children are arrested for drug offenses. Nearly eight thousand teenagers, every day, become sexually active. Six hundred teens get a sexually transmitted disease. One hundred thousand American children are homeless.

These numbers are horrifying. They are staggering. And yet, if you follow the pattern these numbers establish, you will see one thing: most of these problems are related to health—Social health, Medical health, Health knowledge.

Health professionals have worked together in the past to slay the dragons that crippled and robbed young lives—Rickets, Polio, Whooping cough. These are killers that we whipped in another generation. Teenage pregnancy is the polio of this generation. Inadequate prenatal care and crumbling families are the rickets that twist young limbs and rob young minds of their changes. There are our dangerous plagues. Vitamin D will not help. Vaccine will not end it. The cures will be more subtle, more difficult, more time consuming.

I do not suggest that all the social ills of the modern era be dumped on the doorstep of nursing because they are all in your backyard. I suggest only that we must seek heroes who have the expertise and the power to right the wrongs.

All American children deserve the basics of a healthy life. They deserve the fruits of our abundance and the benefits of our pride. Yet, the proportion of United States children in poverty grew by one-third from 1973 to 1988. In that same time period, the United States gross national product grew 47 percent.

It is no longer enough to be caregivers and teachers. We must be advocates. All of us who have the skills and the voices must lend those voices to this struggle.

In recent weeks, I have done a great deal of reading about the curriculum revolution in nursing. I have been inspired by the thoughtful insights into the relationship between knowing and doing. I have been moved by the way the leaders of this profession have incorporated talk and experience into their plan to transform the institutions in which they practice: by the great awareness of the need to go beyond a narrow biomedical perspective to combat the roots of disease such as poverty, homelessness, prejudice, and disadvantage. That is why coming before you to ask for your help in fighting the crusade of the 21st century does not feel presumptuous. Nurses are the agents and leaders for health in our society. That means they also are among the primary agents for educational success, job capability, social productivity, and able parenting—because all these things are by-products of a healthy life beginning at birth.

We have tried to change the world from the top down. We have tried increasing the might of our wealthiest and most advantaged in the hope that the benefits would trickle down to the least advantaged. It did not work. Now we must turn that philosophy on end and try building our national profile from the bottom up. We must give our poorest children the front-end load they deserve, and we will all benefit from their strength.

Not long ago, Harold Shapiro, who is president of Princeton University, talked about the fairy tales of childhood. Goldilocks and Little Red Riding Hood meet up with strangers in the forest. Good ones and bad ones. Dorothy is swept away to Oz and threatened by all kinds of danger. There is always a sense of danger in childhood. You have no power. You worry. Even loved, well-fed children, with predictable lives, worry a great deal. They worry about childhood ending, about neglect and loss of love. Poor children, or those from broken or terribly dysfunctional families, have fears that are greatly magnified. The fear becomes life itself. Not the occasional crisis. Life itself is a scary movie.

You know what would happen if American life was a fairy tale. In fairy tales everyone always gets saved at the last minute. The thing that saves everyone, in every fairy tale, is the benevolent interference of a caring adult. It is time for the good witch to show up. The kindly woodcutter. The fairy godmother. The influence of the caring adult can restore a child's sense of worth, competence, and safety. It can restore innocence where innocence has been stolen. The caring adult provides the child at risk with the safety a child needs to become a useful, happy member of society. One caring adult can make a great deal of difference. Many caring adults working together can make all the difference.

But who will slay the dragon of disadvantage? Who will step in with the wand, the ruby slippers, the handful of magic beans? It will not be one individual. Not one profession. Not one tower of vision. It must be a consortium of professions, a combined vision of many different parts and different life stories. Corporate leaders. Politicians. Teachers. Leaders of the nursing profession. Yes, very importantly, nurses, whose profession is not just a career but a lifework, not just a vocation but a calling. Who have one foot high on the crystal tower of knowledge and theory and one foot in the dust and grit of human need. Nursing professionals, who have a tradition of going not just where the money is but where the need is. Who go home when the job is done, not when the day is done.

It is too much to ask. Yet, there is no one more logical to turn to. You have set the course yourselves, in your bold look at the way you teach your students, in your efforts to establish a national health policy. You have made it clear where you are going to put your political might and your know-how. Nursing professionals will be among the gallant knights, the fairy godmothers and godfathers, the brave champions for our lost children. They will restore the dreams of thousands whose dreams are dying, will rescue the promise of a whole generation. This is the importance of your efforts to shape a health care agenda—nursing's agenda.

Because of the efforts of those here today, a generation of nurses is being trained who will not only treat the diseases of individuals but the diseases of a society. They will understand intimately that their profession means a commitment to the social changes that are necessary for good health, personal and cultural. They will be not only staff nurses, nurse researchers, nurse administrators, nurse educators, and nurse practitioners, but nurse warriors. And, you here, in this audience, will be the Norman Schwartzkopfs of your profession. The generals. The role models and inspirations.

You will be the ones who draw the line in the sand and say, this is where it begins, with this generation.

Such efforts will require all your salesmanship.
Such efforts will require all your creativity.
Such efforts will require all your eloquence.
Such efforts will require all your tolerance and compassion.
Such efforts will require all your toughness and wisdom.

I say all of us, because I am not the one standing here today to make this charge, make it to the leaders of a profession already struggling with many demands and many burdens. I am only the one saying the words.

I'm a teacher, like many of you, whose job right now is leading a great university. But first and foremost, I am an educator, and this charge is directed as much to me and every teacher—of nursing, law, chemistry, economics, and second grade.

I do not issue this challenge. History does. The history of a great nation, revealed by its tradition. I am taking my place beside you, as a warrior, as someone who hopes to be a champion, as someone struggling to answer the most urgent question history has asked in this century.

Will we save our poorest children?

History will only thank us if we have the courage to say yes. If we save our poorest children, we will save our nation. Let's begin together. Let us choose to be heroes. Let your deliberations reflect such courses.

PART TWO

Trends in Nursing Education

2

Recent Trends in Nursing Education

Peri Rosenfeld

*T*he recent, and happily fading, decline in nursing school enrollments and the general concern over the nursing shortage has resulted in renewed attention in data collection and research on nurses. This growing interest, while flattering to researchers, has ironically brought about some unexpected outcomes.

There is a pervasive misunderstanding about the methodological difficulties surrounding data collection. The prevailing attitude seems to be that anybody can construct a survey and collect data on nurses. Nothing could be further from the truth. Nursing education, with its various points of entry, ladders, and exits, is a most challenging area in which to collect data. Consequently, one of the primary functions of the Interagency Conference on Nursing Statistics (ICONS) is to assist in the design of methodological protocols necessary to ensure reliable and valid data on nurses so that the data can be utilized with confidence. In this chapter, I address research design issues related to collecting reliable and valid data, the only viable data to use when formulating policy.

Related to the proliferation of data is the development of information anxiety, a disorienting syndrome caused by the overwhelming bombardment of survey findings, research reports, data elements, and so forth. Victims of information anxiety often find it increasingly difficult to assess and evaluate the utility of the information continually assaulting them. In the final analysis, individuals become weary, unconvinced, and down-right apathetic. Other sufferers of this disorder have the opposite reaction, becoming obsessed with data, requiring empirical proof for every detail.

Hardly, a day goes by without a call from someone asking for obscure data on nurses' life-styles and habits. Often these inquiries involve deep ideological and theoretical justifications. For example, can we truly understand nursing if we do not collect data on leisure activities of newly licensed nurses?

It is important to note that data on nursing education are, relatively speaking, plentiful. In the wake of the nursing shortage, Project Hope (in contract with the Division of Nursing of the U.S. Department of Health and Human Services) reviewed and evaluated available data sources specific to the supply and demand of nurses. The final report identified major data gaps and proposed a timetable for the collection of data necessary to track the supply and demand of nurses. Moreover, the report remarked that, unlike areas such as demand for nurses in nonhospital settings, the National League for Nursing (NLN) and the American Association of Colleges of Nursing (AACN) cover satisfactorily statistics on nurses. The NLN annually collects data on all licensed practical nurses, licensed vocational nurses, registered nurses, and graduate nursing programs and their students. The NLN, in addition, conducts a census of nurse faculty biennially on even years. The American Association of Colleges of Nursing also conducts annual surveys, but concentrates on its membership at the baccalaureate and higher degree level. I focus, in this chapter, on NLN data and will introduce AACN data when appropriate.

Student statistics are helpful in understanding trends related to the future supply of nurses. Nevertheless, it is critical to keep in mind that new graduates represent a fraction of the total supply of nurses. Findings from the 1990 annual survey (National League for Nursing, 1991) reveal that all types of nursing programs are enjoying increased admissions, enrollments, and graduations. Annual admissions to the 1989–90 school year reached over 110,000 bringing the number of new students to its 1980–81 level (Figure 1). Annual admissions peaked in 1983–84 and then fell to a low of 90,000 in 1986–87. The 1990 figure marks the third year of upward progress. Note that all program types reported gains in admissions and that associate degree programs have hit a new high (almost 70,000) in new admissions in 1990.

The enrollment picture is also quite encouraging (Figure 2). In the final analysis, almost 225,000 basic nursing students were enrolled in the nation's nursing schools on October 15, 1990. This 12 percent jump over the 1989 figure reflects healthy gains in all program types. Diploma programs report their first increase in enrollments since 1981 and associate degree enrollments reached an all-time high of almost 120,000 in Fall 1990.

Graduations, ostensibly the most important statistic for understanding the nursing supply, surged 9 percent to just over 67,000 in 1990 (Figure 3). While still distant from the 1985 peak of 82,000, this figure represents the first year of improvement since the downward trend

Recent Trends in Nursing Education

FIGURE 1
Ten-Year Trend in Annual Admissions

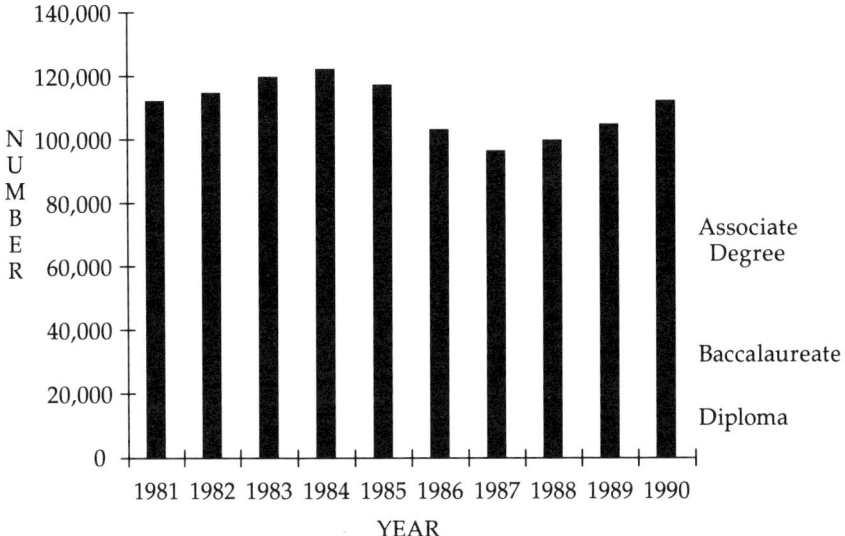

Note: From 1990 Annual Survey of Nursing Education, National League for Nursing, Division of Research.

FIGURE 2
Ten-Year Trend in Enrollments

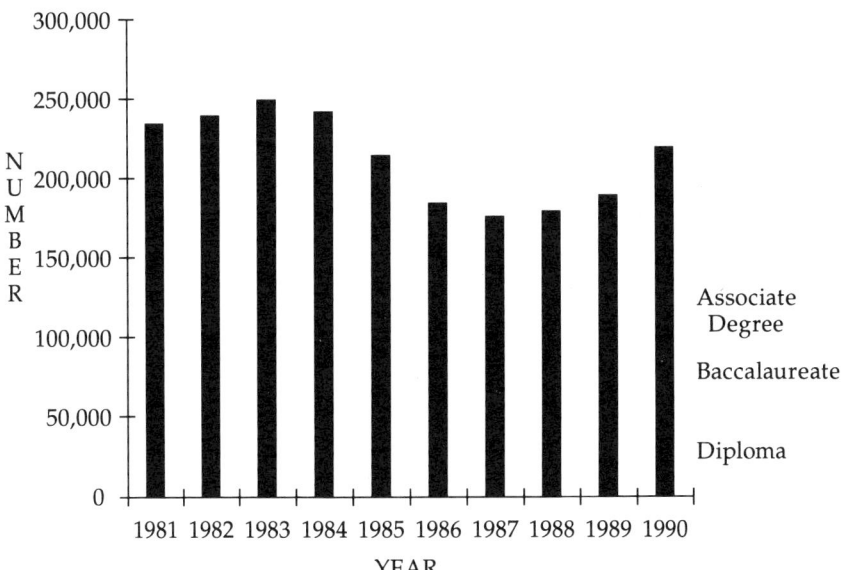

Note: From 1990 Annual Survey of Nursing Education, National League for Nursing, Division of Research.

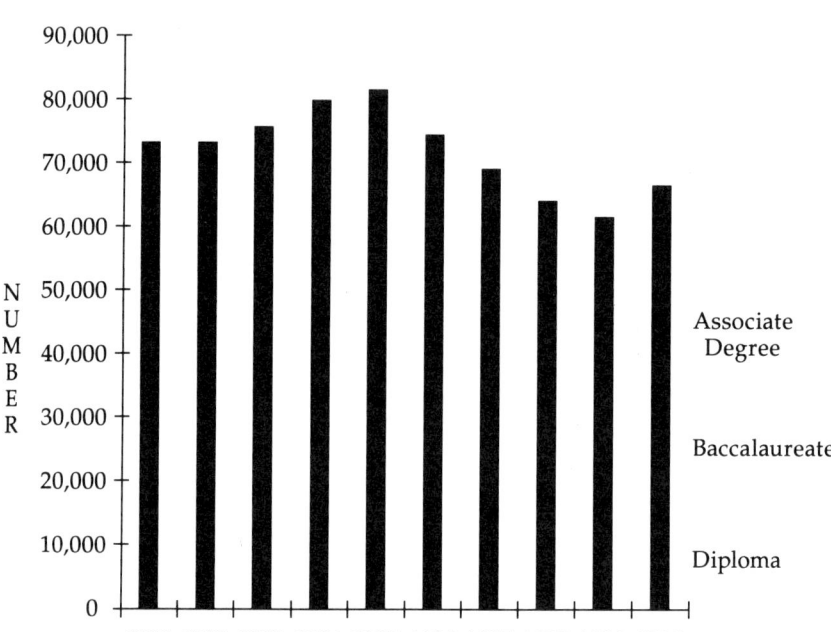

FIGURE 3
Ten-Year Trend in Graduations

Note: From 1990 Annual Survey of Nursing Education, National League for Nursing, Division of Research.

begun in 1986. All program types reported improvements, with associate degree programs leading the pack. The complete findings on registered nurses will appear in the NLN's *Nursing DataSource 1991, Vol. 1.*

The renewed interest in nursing has important implications for the institutions and faculties that prepare nurses for their professional careers. Specifically, the question arises, are there and will there be sufficient numbers of qualified faculty to prepare the growing number of students interested in pursuing nursing? Recently released data from the 1990 census of faculty (*Nurse Educator,* 1991) explores these issues. These data monitor trends in the number and characteristics of nurse faculty members and track their credentials, workloads, and salaries.

A recent press release from AACN reported that about 16 percent of the responding baccalaureate programs could not accept qualified students. Of those 79 programs which had to reject qualified students, half claimed that faculty shortages were to blame. These data are tempting, but let me put them into perspective. First, a relatively small number of schools claim shortages—16 percent does not constitute a crisis. In addition, there is the problem of using a subjective definition for measuring shortages. Then, how do we examine objectively the issue of faculty shortages? Traditionally, a shortage exists when an inordinate number of budgeted vacant positions remain unfilled in spite of active recruitment. In this sense, a faculty shortage is not evident according to the 1990 findings that report the existence of fewer than 800 vacant faculty positions. This is equivalent to a 5 percent vacancy rate among the nation's nursing schools. This figure, while disconcerting, is certainly not unusual or alarming.

Vacancy rates, however, are not a sufficient measure of shortages for a variety of reasons. Most importantly, they are based on an employer or budget perspective (i.e., the administrator's assessment of either the requisite number of faculty necessary to educate students or the number of faculty they can afford). This administrative assessment may be conservative in regard to economic circumstances, educational philosophy, and local market conditions. One important lesson learned from the Secretary's Commission (1988) and the Project Hope report involved the limited utility of vacancy rates in evaluating the recent nursing shortages in the nation's hospitals. So, if vacancy rates are not infallible, what other data exist to speak to the issue of faculty shortages? Faculty census data clearly reveal that the number of full-time faculty has remained fairly stagnant since 1986 (Figure 4) and

FIGURE 4
Trends in Full-Time Faculty, 1980–1990

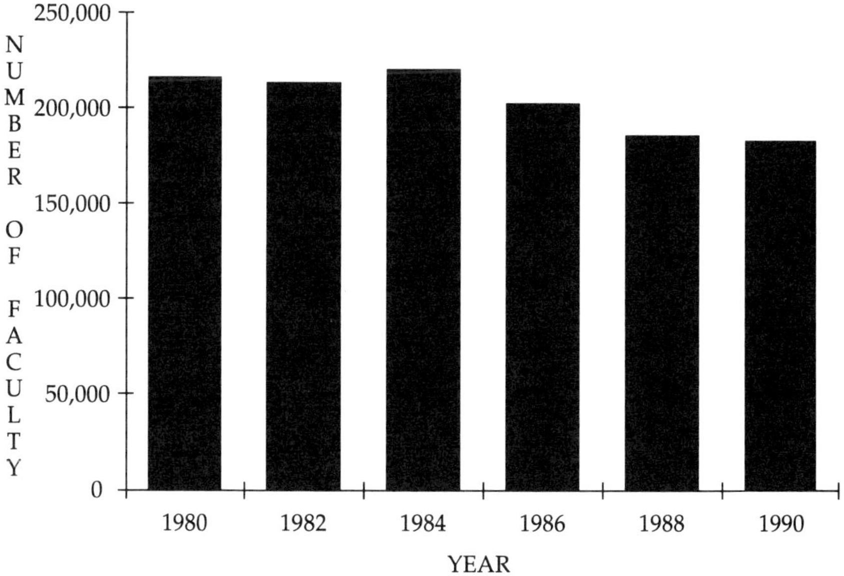

Note: From *Nurse Educator: Findings from the Faculty Census,* National League for Nursing, Division of Research, 1991.

that the number of vacant positions appears fairly static since 1988 despite the increasing number of students flocking to the nation's schools of nursing (Figure 5). On the other hand, the use of part-time faculty is increasing dramatically (Figure 6). This suggests that schools of nursing are not expanding their slots for full-time faculty and are opting to hire part-timers.

Most colleges and universities insist that tenure track, full-time professors attain higher levels of graduate education than part-time faculty. The trend toward part-time employment may be partially explained by the inability to recruit credentialed individuals for full-time faculty. Undoubtedly, there also are economic considerations. Part-timers are less expensive. Also, many are graduate students and are satisfied to be hired as part-time faculty. Upon receipt of their graduate degrees, these part-timers are likely to leave academia for industry, health care, and elsewhere where the opportunities are greater and the salaries higher.

FIGURE 5
Trends in Vacancy Rates, 1980–1990

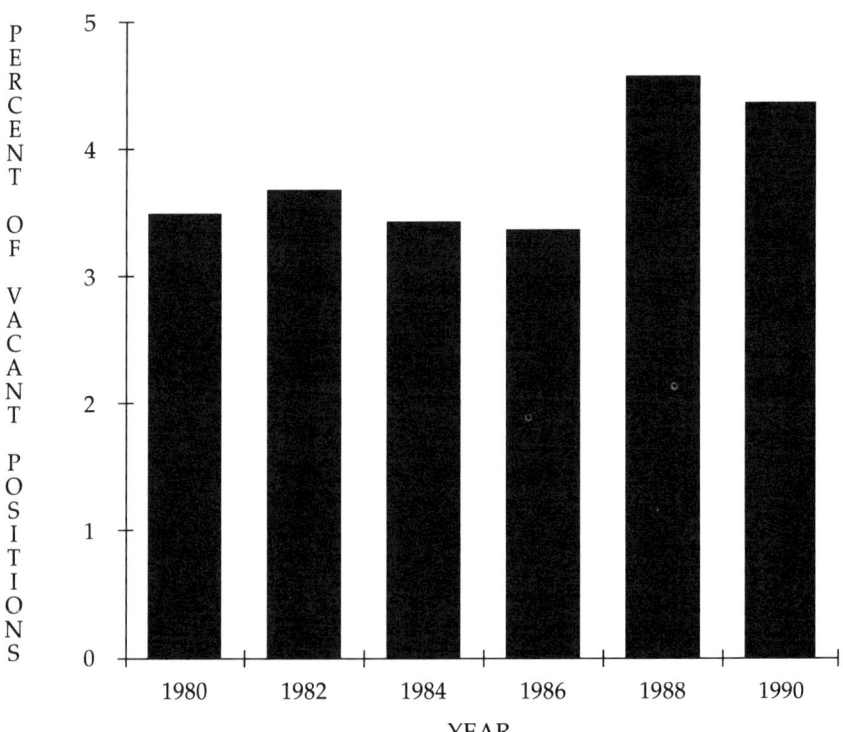

Note: From *Nurse Educator: Findings from the Faculty Census,* National League for Nursing, Division of Research, 1991.

FIGURE 6
Trends in Part-Time Faculty, 1980–1990

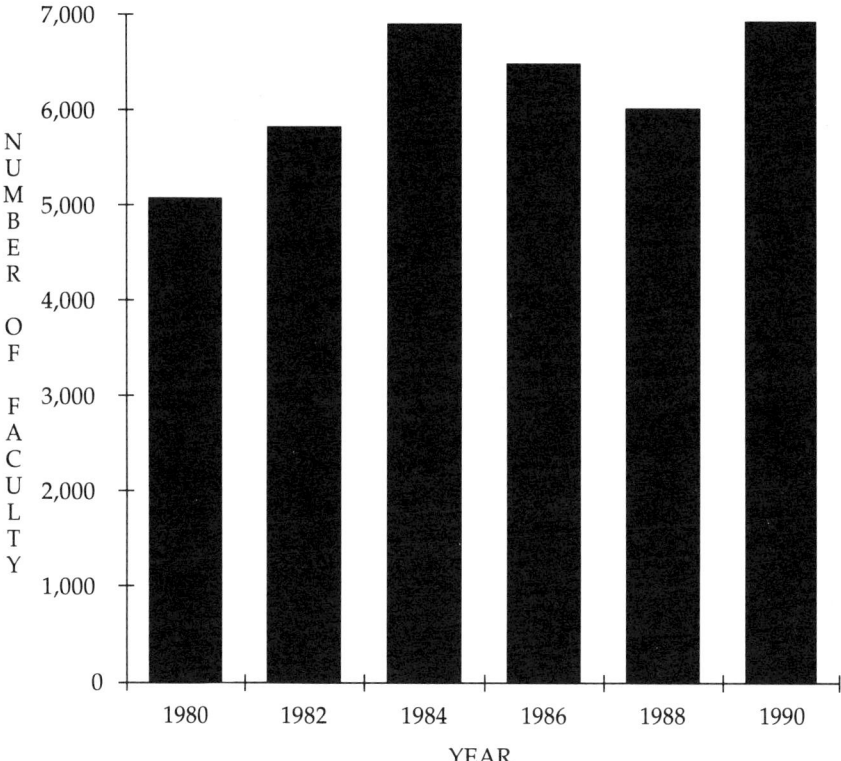

Note: From *Nurse Educator: Findings from the Faculty Census,* National League for Nursing, Division of Research, 1991.

Another explanation is that the decline, in the mid-1980s, in student enrollments forced nursing schools to limit their full-time positions. Meanwhile, the growth in career options for individuals with advanced nursing degrees also affects the competitive edge in institutions of higher learning. As noted in the Division of Nursing's report to Congress, the demand for nurses prepared at the masters and doctoral level is outstripping the supply (Figure 7). Opportunities in areas such as clinical specialties, research, management and administration, business, and peer review and quality assurance are attracting many registered nurses who would otherwise take positions in academia. These nonacademic opportunities are often much more lucrative and have the professional challenges many associate with academia. For example, the average salary of a doctoral-prepared registered nurse in an associate degree program is in the mid-$40,000s. In contrast, the corresponding figure for a graduate-prepared registered nurse in service is near

FIGURE 7
Projected Supply and Demand for RNs Prepared at the Master's/Doctoral Level, 2000

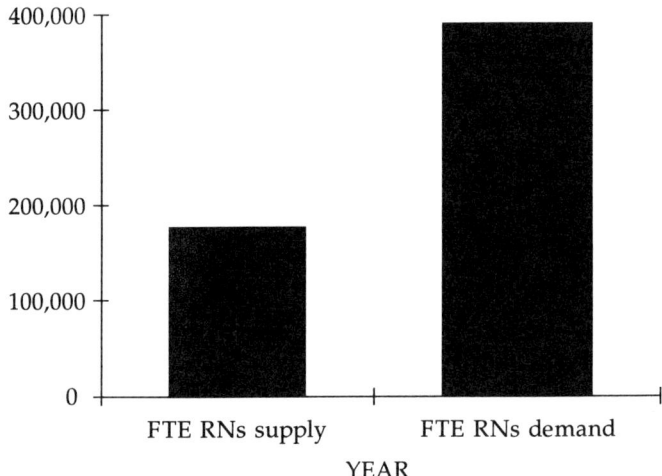

Note: From U.S. Department of Health and Human Services (1990, March). *Seventh Report to Congress.* Washington, DC: Author.

$70,000 and can go as high as $150,000, according to a recent American Organization of Nurse Executives (1990) survey.

The impending shortage of faculty is not unique to nurses. A decade ago, new PhDs glutted the academic market. Thus, many took positions in nonacademic settings such as nonprofit organizations, research, and government. In fact, well-paying nonacademic opportunities grew in business and management for a great part of the 1980s, further eroding the attraction of academia. As a result of these trends, institutions of higher learning are now faced with a dilemma. The number of individuals with the appropriate credentials to teach at collegiate level has shrunk and highly educated candidates are less willing to forgo profitable alternatives for the modest salaries offered at the nation's colleges and universities. While the predicament faced by nursing is not unusual, it requires a uniquely *nursing* resolution. As opportunities expand elsewhere, who will remain to prepare the future cadre of nurses?

REFERENCES

Department of Health and Human Services. (1988). *Secretary's commission on nursing: Final report.* Washington, DC: Author.

National League for Nursing. (1991). *Nursing data source,* Volume I. New York: Author.

National League for Nursing. (1991). *Nurse educator: Findings from the faculty census.* New York: Author.

_____. (1990). Today's nurse executive data analysis survey. AONE & Witt Associates, Inc.

PART THREE

Cultural Diversity in Nursing Education

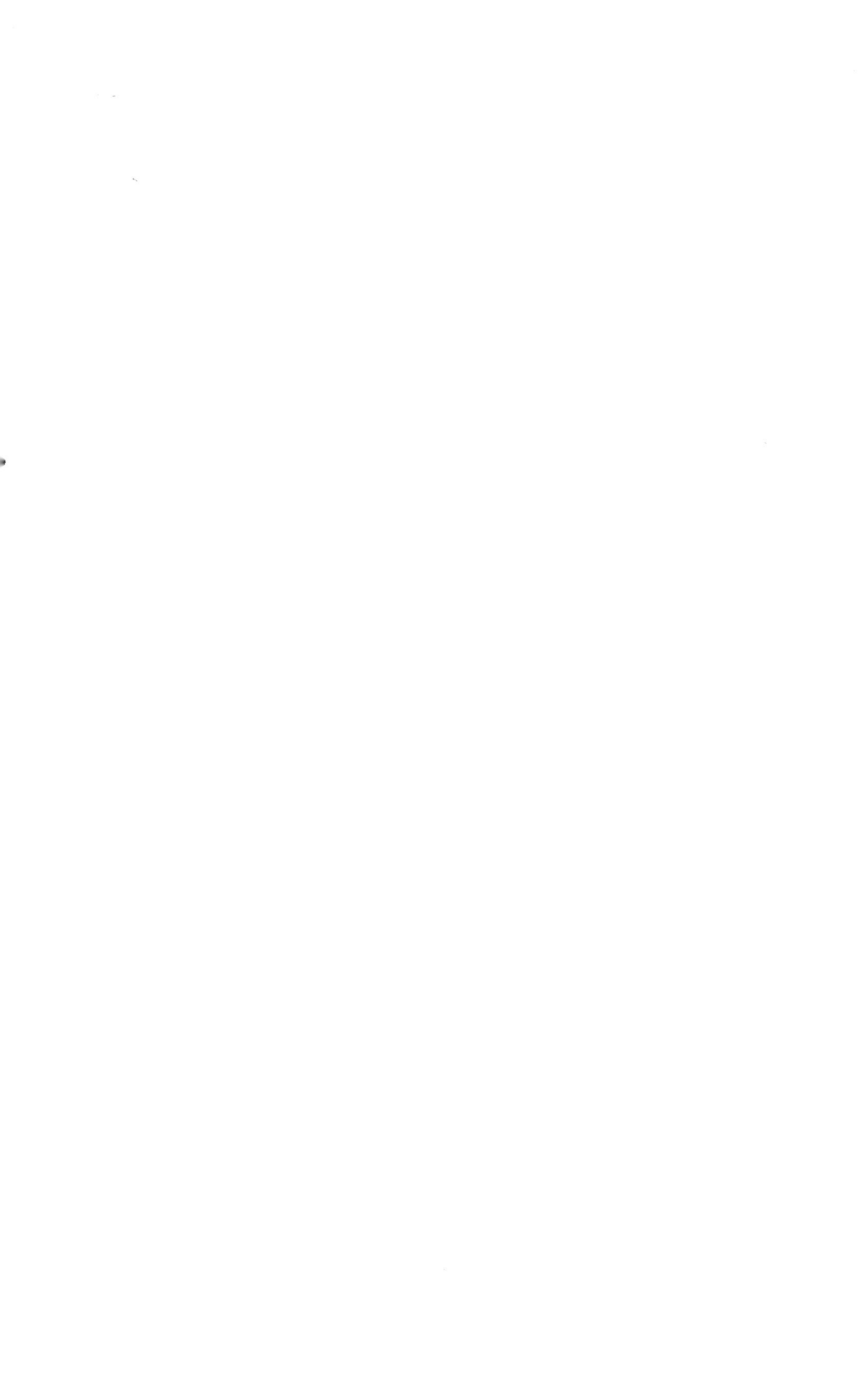

3

Quality Education for Minorities: Myths, Realities, and Strategies

Shirley M. McBay

No topic is more important to our country's future than the well-being of millions of Americans, including more than 48 million African Americans, Alaska Natives, American Indians, Mexican Americans, and Puerto Ricans. Currently, our educational and health care systems underserve low-income families and their children, a group that is disproportionately minority. It is precisely the reality of our educational system that led to the creation of the Quality Education for Minorities Project, based at MIT, and later to the Quality Education for Minorities Network, a nonprofit organization established in July 1990 in Washington, DC. These two organizations are dedicated to improving education for minorities throughout the nation. The Network is a focal point for the implementation of strategies to help realize the vision and goals set forth in the report *Education That Works: An Action Plan for the Education of Minorities* (1990). The report was issued by the Quality Education for Minorities Project, following more than two years of research around the country. We met with hundreds of people about issues related to the education of minorities and visited sites to learn about effective programs and strategies to improve the education of minority children, youth, and adults. In our report, we outlined six major goals and 58 recommendations for ensuring quality education for minorities. We were pleased later to see these six goals reflected in the National Education Goals established by the President and the governors.

In this chapter, I want to examine some of the myths and realities preventing minorities from receiving quality education and quality health care, as well as some of the reasons for their underrepresentation in higher education, specifically in science-based fields, including the health professions. I will suggest several steps that we can take, as individuals or as an organization, to help address the problems that we face as a country and that prevent us from providing quality education for all children.

Minorities are seriously underrepresented among all health care personnel, including nurses, and especially among upper level health administrators. This underrepresentation is particularly serious for blacks and Hispanics in proportion to their overall representation in the general population. The recent seventh report to the President and Congress on the status of health care personnel in the U.S. attributed this underrepresentation to "inadequate educational preparation at the high school level; inadequate or inappropriate career counseling; admissions policies of some health professional schools/programs; relatively high attrition rates after matriculation; and substantial costs of obtaining education as a health professional." While all of these factors are important, there are also others that serve as barriers to minority students entering higher education and science-based fields, including the health-related professions.

Both the traditionally poor health care received by the majority of this nation's minority populations and the barriers to adequate health care for the uninsured millions of American citizens in urban and rural areas (estimated overall at around 32 million) signal a national imperative to increase the number of minority health care personnel in this country. As the seventh report states, "motivation to increase minority representation derives not only from a need to assure equal access to health professions education to all population groups, but from a need for more practitioners to provide health care to minorities and other disadvantaged populations." Recent studies demonstrate that underrepresented minority practitioners are much more likely to locate and practice in medically underserved and poverty areas, a finding that is particularly encouraging for the future as we hopefully intensify our efforts to recruit and retain minority students in health-related fields.

One could argue that by addressing issues inherent in the lack of minority access to quality education, in particular quality mathematics and science education, we can address their underrepresentation in the health professions and access to quality health care. Consider the following four points.

First, we are a nation increasingly dependent on science and technology, particularly on the rapid flow and retrieval of information. As scientific and technological advances enhance our lives in such areas as energy, medicine, and communications, they also present major challenges. For example, by the year 2000 we will have for the first time in our history a majority of new jobs requiring education beyond high school, particularly in the fields of mathematics, science, and engineering. The health professions, including nursing, are themselves increasingly dependent on strong mathematics and science education and training.

Second, there is growing concern about whether the supply of health personnel will be adequate to meet the nation's requirements for health care in the future, particularly after the year 2000. We are a nation in the midst of a crisis within our delivery systems for both health and education. Our health needs in preventive medicine, nutrition, and primary health care delivery are increasing. Our growing aging population demands increasing health care and nursing home services. Increased infant mortality, particularly among minority and immigrant populations, requires greater access to quality pre- and postnatal care. Our nation's increasing problems with substance abuse as well as the crisis of increased AIDS transmission, require significant new health care and social services.

Third, demographic shifts are rapidly transforming our school population and hence our future workforce. Reports such as the Hudson Institute's *Workforce 2000: Work and Workers for the 21st Century* project that 85 percent of the net growth in our workforce for the rest of this century will be met by minorities, women, and immigrants.

Fourth, issues regarding quality education for minorities and minority access to higher education cannot be divorced from the myths about education and about minorities that permeate our society nor can they be separated from issues of socioeconomic status.

Among the myths that help explain why minorities are behind are the following:

- Learning is due to innate ability and minorities are simply less capable of educational excellence than whites.
- The situation is hopeless; the problems minority youth face including poverty, teenage pregnancy, unemployment, substance abuse, and high dropout rates are so overwhelming that society is incapable of providing effective responses.
- Quality education for all is a luxury, since not all jobs presently require creativity and problem-solving skills.
- Education is an expense and not an investment.
- Equity and excellence in education are in conflict.
- All we need are marginal changes.
- Minorities do not care about education.
- Bilingual education delays the learning of English and hinders academic achievement.
- The problem will go away.
- Educational success or failure is within the complete control of each individual; in America anybody can make it.

These myths are pervasive and are sustained by an obsolete, factory model educational system that only produces an educated elite, a group too small to meet the demands of a world class economy. That these myths are alive and well can be seen in the results of a survey conducted by the National Opinion Research Center at the University of Chicago for the National Science Foundation. According to the *Washington Post* of January 9, 1991, "A majority of whites believe blacks and Hispanics are likely to prefer welfare to hard work and tend to be lazier than whites, more prone to violence, less intelligent, and less patriotic." More specifically, according to the *Post* article, 53 percent of whites in the survey said they think blacks are less intelligent than whites and 55 percent thought Hispanics were less intelligent than whites. Such myths prevent the country from dealing with its seriously outmoded educational system.

It is not clear that mainstream America really knows and understands the implications of holding on to an educational system whose graduates by and large do not have the ability to solve complex problems, to analyze abstract knowledge, to communicate with precision, to deal with change and ambiguity, and to work well with other people, especially those from diverse cultures and backgrounds. Otherwise, would it not be obvious that it is not in our national interest to hold on to a system that produces such graduates, that disproportionately places low-income and minority children and youth into lower track classes where they are most often taught in a climate of low expectations, by the least experienced teachers, and with the fewest resources? Would we knowingly give these students, upon whom our domestic and military security will increasingly depend, less of everything they need to be successful? Are our myths blinding us to the demographic and workforce realities? To the injustice and immorality of our system?

In addition to the myths about education and about minorities, there are other obstacles to quality education in and out of school. These include: inadequate school financing; too few minority teachers; overreliance on testing; poorly prepared teachers; disregard of language and cultural diversity; absence of an educational legacy in one's family or community; negative peer pressure; and of course, poverty and hopelessness.

Poverty in our cities, especially among children, is increasing in tragic proportions. In a recent report detailing the erosion of school-age children's well-being during the 1980s, the Center for the Study of Social Policy reported that the percentage of black children in 1990 living in poverty was 43.8 percent; for Hispanic children, the poverty rate was 38.2 percent; and the rate for white children was 15.4 percent. I need not remind the reader how closely poverty is related to inadequate nutrition, health and family care, and housing; nor how these factors, in turn, help explain school dropouts and school failure.

Our school age population is increasingly minority, immigrant, and poor. We are a country seeking to survive in an increasingly competitive global economy and in need of a workforce with higher level skills throughout, not simply at the top. Ironically, to meet our workforce needs, including in the health care fields, America must turn to the very groups whose education and health needs it has so grossly neglected in the past.

In short, America must reach out in new and more effective ways to encourage and enable minority students to enter college in significant numbers prepared to be successful and not in need of remedial assistance. Once in college, they must find supportive and hospitable environments in which to study. Minority college graduates, who have successfully studied mathematics and science, must not only have science and health careers as realistic career options, but must be able to move upward through the ranks of their profession. As in college and graduate or professional school, they must have mentors in the workplace who can help them succeed. Why are these outcomes so difficult to achieve? Why, in light of all we know about what is necessary for academic and workplace success, are minority students unable to enter into college and into science-based careers in ever larger numbers? The answers to these questions, in my view, lie first and foremost in our ability, as individuals, as communities, as organizations, and as a country, to come to terms with our myths, the institutionalized racism inherent in our educational system, and the racial hatred and stereotypes embedded in far too many of our hearts.

We must have the individual and national will to make the long-term commitment required to solve the racial problems we face. There are other places to look as well. The answers to increased access to higher education also lie in our ability to focus attention and strategies in a holistic and coordinated way from prenatal to the graduate or professional stage. Let me briefly comment on some of these stages.

PRE- AND POSTNATAL

Many people mistakenly believe that issues relating to education begin at preschool; however, attention must be focused much earlier if all children are to begin school prepared to learn. In this country, over 5 million children—one child in four—are born into poverty and the number is growing at alarming rates. In 1987, about 2.1 million or 42 percent of 5 million poor children under six were white, about 1.6 million or 32 percent were black, 1 million or 21 percent were Hispanic, and another 5 percent, 250,000, were American Indians, Asians, and other racial or ethnic backgrounds. Given their disproportionate representation among the poor, it should not be surprising then that blacks, Hispanics, and American Indians comprise the groups that are traditionally the most underserved by our health care system and our educational system.

The connection between poverty, poor health, and low educational achievement is evident and the policy implications are clear. We know how much difference quality pre- and postnatal care can mean for birth weight, life expectancy, and early health development of children; and we know too the connection between poverty, poor health, and poor nutrition of mothers and the readiness of their young children for school.

A research and policy review of health programs for poor young children issued by the National Center for Children in Poverty documents the close relationship between poverty and children's health problems, demonstrating how economic hardship, social circumstances, and inadequate health service delivery work together to engender in the poor "despair and powerlessness that hinder healthy behavior." According to the report, "poor children are more likely than non poor children to be born too soon or too small; to die in the first year of life; to experience acute illness, injuries, lead poisoning, child abuse, and neglect; and to suffer from nutrition-related problems and chronic illnesses—many of which are preventable." Interestingly enough, the report concludes that "when financial barriers are removed, the care-seeking behavior of many of the poor closely resembles that of the non poor." The intricate tie between socioeconomic status, poor health, and poor educational achievement could not be more clearly stated than in this report.

Poverty and lack of health care, as well as the absence, for most poor children, of early intervention programs such as Head Start result in a poor child entering school considerably behind the child born into a more affluent family. The disparity is so large that the equal opportunity public schooling should provide becomes a cruel hoax, because in actuality there is no level playing field from the very beginning nor does it ever become level for the majority of these youngsters. Our system of public education should allow each child an equal opportunity to succeed, but this opportunity never begins for many children; almost inevitably and often knowingly, the poor minority child is left behind.

PRESCHOOL

At the preschool level, however, we can point to the tremendous success of the Head Start program that was started in 1965. Through its four components of Education, Health Care, Parental Involvement, and Social Services, Head Start has proven that it makes a difference in people's lives and gives children the chance to begin school ready to learn. The problem, however, is that Head Start only reaches 20 percent of the children eligible for it. Similarly, the Women, Infant, and Children Program (WIC), "the special supplemental food program for women, infants, and children" reaches only half of those eligible for it. It is because of the critical importance of these early stages of development—from prenatal through preschool—that the Quality Education for Minorities' first goal states, "We must ensure that minority students start school prepared to learn."

ELEMENTARY AND MIDDLE HIGH SCHOOL

The critical years of elementary and middle high school, the third stage, gives me the opportunity to address some of the issues surrounding the public school system in this country which most minority children attend. For most minority children, school means a hierarchical, educational system that discourages, rather than promotes, quality education, especially for students from low socioeconomic backgrounds. These students, often as early as kindergarten, are disproportionately relegated to low track classes in such critical subjects as reading and mathematics, groupings from which they seldom recover. In our elementary and middle schools, we find the majority of minority children already labeled as "slow learners." They have been and are disproportionately placed in low track classes where they are taught to memorize, through drill and practice, by the least experienced teachers, with the fewest resources, and in a climate of low expectations. In the meantime, our "factory model system" of public education treats more affluent students as gifted and talented, holds high expectations of them, and provides them with the very best teachers.

In most cases, because of preschool and out-of-school enriching experiences that derive from their more privileged backgrounds and because they have been singled out along with a small group of peers with similar backgrounds for an academically challenging and rewarding experience, these children feel special and their self-esteem is high. It is often these students who are strong in mathematics and science and who assume from an early age that they will go to college.

HIGH SCHOOL

The fourth stage—high school—has its own challenges for students wishing to enter the professions. It is in high school that students must complete a strong academic core curriculum if they are to be prepared for success in college. Nevertheless, it is also in high school that the crippling effects of tracking in the lower grades become even more evident. For example, most low tracked students do not get to take such college gatekeeper courses as algebra and geometry. If they do, it is well into high school and too late for them to take other higher level mathematics and science courses they will need to have science-based careers as realistic options.

In the public schools, the debilitating practice of tracking must be eliminated and an environment that is conducive for success for all students must be created. This environment would be created by largely restructured schools having as their hallmarks the following characteristics:

- A strong core curriculum
- Competent and motivated teachers
- Extensive parental and community involvement
- Effective and innovative teaching strategies
- Access to state of the art instructional technology
- Year-round enrichment
- Systematic assessment of student progress
- Systematic exposure to career options
- Special emphasis on mathematics and science
- A supportive and caring environment

A high school with these characteristics would prepare students for success in college or the workplace and would enable more students, including minority students, to have science-based careers as realistic options. In addition, if more high schools were to provide health professions internships and community service opportunities, it is more likely that larger numbers of students would see health fields as viable career alternatives. One of the encouraging recent developments is the establishment of comprehensive school health education programs. In such situations, health and social services are provided on site and instruction offered on disease prevention, nutrition, and sound life behaviors. Such programs also contribute to healthier and safer school environments. Through community health centers in schools and training for early parenting associated with child care facilities, schools have the opportunity to help in the delivery of services that can begin to deal with the inextricable connections between poverty, poor health, poor nutrition, and low educational achievement.

Quality Education for Minorities is encouraging such community-based comprehensive centers not only in schools, but in housing developments and geographically low-income residential communities. Such a model would focus and coordinate resources and support services of federal, state, and local agencies, community-based organizations, churches, colleges, universities, and other community groups in a position to provide educational, social, health, and housing services in low-income communities. This holistic service delivery model, which would concentrate resources in a defined community, would focus on school readiness and on the education of minority children and youth beginning with prenatal health care, thus enabling families to better assume their roles and responsibilities as parents.

I want to briefly comment on the tremendous difficulties minority students often face in completing college and graduate or professional school. First among these issues is, of course, financial aid. Minority students are most likely to come from low-income families who have little or no resources to help their children gain a college education. In addition, inadequate preparation for college forces many minority students to enroll in remedial courses. Thus, for reasons of finance, academic preparation, and lack of encouragement, these students are seldom able to take advantage of other enriching opportunities in college, for example, community service opportunities that increase commitment to education and provide motivation to stay in school and to serve as role models for other students in the community.

But why should we really worry about all of this? Why should we change? Let me give you four good reasons.

1. *Moral:* Our factory model educational system, with its practice of tracking, perpetuates the myths of white superiority and of the innate inferiority of certain minorities. It legitimizes lower expectations of minorities and makes it the norm. Under it, we continue to knowingly give low socioeconomic status minority children less of everything that we know is necessary for success and then blame them when they don't succeed.

2. *Demographic:* The country is becoming increasingly minority and hence increasingly dependent upon the very groups most underserved by our educational system, those most prevalently found in the lower tracks from preschool to college.

3. *Economic:* The country cannot get by with just an educated elite. We need a quality workforce throughout.

4. *Our ideals as a nation:* We cannot afford to have the majority of our young people with low self-esteem and a second-rate education. What we have created runs counter to our ideal as a land of equal opportunity for all.

By restructuring our educational system and eliminating tracking, we reduce truancy and dropouts; we increase self-esteem and confidence; we save millions of dollars invested to study why students drop out and to finance after-the-fact programs; we reduce the need for business and industry to spend billions of dollars in retraining;

we recover the costs of lost income from potential earnings and from lower productivity; and we reduce the likelihood of increased crime and of yet another generation of parents with low self-esteem, few skills, and untapped talent.

Finally, what can you do to help improve the quality of education that minority children and youth receive? You can work with local school systems to ensure that health education becomes an integral part of the curriculum at least by the third grade. You can push for on-site health clinics or health referral services so that low-income children and their families have the knowledge and the access they need to secure quality health care. You can become involved in your community's school reform efforts; you can insist, for example, that educational strategies such as cooperative learning and group projects are systematically used beginning in the early grades. You can encourage your local school board to begin, for example, to require all students to take algebra in the middle school, thereby increasing their likelihood of enrolling in college preparatory mathematics and science courses and of later attending and succeeding in college. You can participate in school and community efforts or serve as a mentor all along the educational continuum to help make clearer to students the connection between what is happening in the classroom and everyday life. You can help strengthen the bonds between local schools and the community. You can help form alliances and partnerships involving parents, community-based organizations, social service agencies, and local businesses by helping to persuade them that change is possible if individuals and groups are motivated to act and to work together to meet common goals and objectives.

You can help create a plan for your community's school that:

- Ensures that every child in your community starts school prepared to learn (e.g., through full funding of Head Start and WIC)
- Develops clear expectations of students and of parents
- Stimulates and nourishes positive values

Such a plan can lead to schools whose graduates:

- Appreciate the intrinsic joy of learning
- Know the pleasure of using their minds to solve problems and come up with ideas
- Know the self-satisfaction and pleasure of doing a project well
- Appreciate and respect their own accomplishments as well as those of others
- Appreciate the importance of the role of the family in their lives

- Are willing to work with others toward a common objective
- Have the self-confidence to make decisions based on their own ideas and experiences
- Respect points of view that may be different from their own
- Accept people different from themselves and have a genuine interest in learning about other cultures
- Take responsibility for doing things that need to be done and do them well, from beginning to end
- Understand that helping others is both a responsibility and its own reward
- Have a commitment to honesty, truth, and self-discipline
- Understand that learning is a life-long process and the best way to have the most control over one's life

There is no doubt that each of you can help to provide the leadership needed at the community level and within national organizations to which you belong. You can help to develop the strategies and the support needed to meet the challenges facing our public schools and our country and preventing untold numbers of talented low-income students from experiencing academic success and fulfillment. To not act is to risk the country's domestic security. The task before us is clear. We must put an end to the educational neglect of low-income and minority children. We can begin by eliminating tracking, by holding high expectations of all children and youth, and by developing partnerships within our respective communities to generate the broadbased support needed for the radical changes we seek.

Ending the neglect of these young people is part of the answer to America's larger problems. The road to the future must be paved with the achievements of all of our children and not just a privileged few. We must seek to build an America where no one is left out. We must do so not only because it is right, although that is reason enough, but because the future well-being and economic security of our communities and our country depend upon it. Despite its frequent failure to live up to its highest aspirations, the greatness of America has always derived from its ability to blend the strengths of very different kinds of people. America has succeeded because at every turn it has been able to bring its most precious natural resource to bear on the tasks at hand: a diverse and talented people. In the twentieth century, it has been the slow maturation of the nation's pluralism, the growing recognition that every current in the American stream teems with new life and greater possibility, that has expanded our reach and enriched our lives. The one force that has sustained and empowered all our people has been the power of education. It has been our schools that have equipped individuals to transform visions into realities and to translate lofty goals into tasks that could be grasped and achieved. Minority children, by right and by virtue of their unlimited potential, surely deserve their own role as visionaries, as builders, and as future leaders. It is in our classrooms, our schools, and our community health centers and health maintenance organizations that the economic future of the nation will be determined. We look to the health professionals to provide and inspire the delivery of quality health care. We look to the schools to provide the educated citizenry and the skilled workforce that America needs to sustain itself.

4

Diversity in Nursing Faculty Hinges on Diversity in Nursing Students

Sallie Tucker-Allen

*I*n this chapter I want to address cultural diversity from both a faculty and student perspective. I base this on my experience as a faculty member for the past twenty years, results obtained from research focusing on both minority students and black faculty members, and a literature review.

NURSING AND THE HEALTH CARE COMPLEX

Over a 24-year period, the health care industry has grown by 292 percent, currently employing 6 million workers within its ranks. This explosive growth means that health care makes up 11 percent of the gross national product of the United States. This means that close to one out of every ten dollars is spent on health care; a fact that makes health care a central spoke in the United States' economic wheel. What importance does this fact have for nursing and for schools of nursing?

First, even though the health care industry is in a boom phase, health care is not being equitably distributed throughout American communities. Large segments of the population are denied access or lack access to health care providers and services. These persons include, but are not limited to the poor, the unemployed, the uninsured, the underinsured, the homeless, and those residing in both large urban areas as well as geographically remote areas. This is exacerbated as the American economy moves toward a part-time workforce where health insurance is not included in the employment package. Second, an inequitable number of those lacking access to health care are minorities. Even when minorities can access the health care system they may find few minority nurses with whom they can identify. Nursing is still a predominantly white, middle-class, female profession. Third, data reported by the American Association of Colleges of Nursing, (1991) show that, though minorities represent nearly 20 percent of the United States population, they comprise only 7 percent of the 2 million registered nurses. Furthermore, overall enrollments have recently increased in schools of nursing, while the percentage of minority students has remained almost unchanged at 17.1 percent during 1990–91. Of this number, blacks comprise 10.6 percent, Asian Pacific Islanders total 3.2 percent, Hispanics stand at 2.8 percent and Native Americans at 0.5 percent. Fourth, with the recent increase in the number of students admitted to schools of nursing, it has been projected that there looms a shortage of nursing faculty members ("Big Gains," 1990). This shortage will not only affect nursing but with the graying of faculty members, a concomitant universitywide shortage of faculty has been projected by the year 2000. In addition, it has been projected that within the early part of the next century, the majority of citizens in the United States will be of minority status.

Consequently, one can expect that universities and nursing schools will experience an overall shortage of faculty members, and that the number of students matriculating in both universities and schools of nursing will include a larger number of minorities. What is it that faculty members need to know in order to teach and work effectively with this new cohort?

FEMALES IN HIGHER EDUCATION

To work more effectively with the new students entering nursing, faculty members of all racial and ethnic groups need to understand the relationship which has historically existed between males and females in this country. For example, data reveal that in 1986–87 women received 40 percent of all PhD degrees granted from institutions of higher education. Of this number, minorities received 11 percent. In 1987–88, women held only 27 percent of all faculty positions, with minorities holding 10 percent of them. It has been suggested that the revolving door syndrome is the primary reason for the lack of increase in the numbers of women and minorities in higher education. Moses (1989) reported that blacks have the lowest faculty retention and promotion rates in academia. A similar finding was made by the University of Wisconsin Regents who noted that minority women have the highest departure rate in the University of Wisconsin System, followed by nonminority women, and then by minority males. Diversity is, therefore, not just a concept related specifically to nursing faculty, but is a concept which should be viewed from a universitywide perspective.

In looking at diversity from this perspective, we need to look at the broader concept of women in higher education. In 1982, Hall and Sandler noted that women are the new majority on American campuses and that their education has become central to the survival of the postsecondary enterprise.

Within the university environment, however, subtle forms of discrimination take place, affecting how women view themselves and how much they achieve. For example, male professors may devalue female colleagues, their work, and accomplishments. Male professors may expect less of female students, frown on feminine behavior, and overtly display sexist verbal behavior toward female students. Hall and Sandler (1982) feel that these small differences can "create an environment which maintains unequal opportunity and inequity" (p. 5). Examples of nonverbal behavior of male professors shaping the classroom climate include: making eye contact with men more often than with women students, nodding and gesturing more often in response to men's questions and comments than to women's, using a modulating tone with female students, excluding women from course-related activities, grouping students according to sex, favoring men in choosing student assistants, and making direct sexual overtures to female students.

Male faculty behaviors which may promote student invisibility include: ignoring women students while recognizing male students, calling directly on male students but not on female students, calling male students by name more often than women students, addressing the class as if no women were present, coaching male students but not female students toward a fuller answer, waiting longer for males than for females to answer a question before going on to another student, interrupting women students or allowing them to be disproportionately interrupted by peers, asking men students questions that require a higher order of thinking, responding more extensively to male's questions than to women's comments, phrasing classroom examples in a way which reinforces a stereotyped and negative view of women's psychological traits.

By inserting blacks and other minorities in the examples listed above one can see how these same behaviors apply to minority students. For example, white nursing faculty may make more eye contact with white nursing students than black students. They may nod and gesture more often in response to comments from white students than from black students. They may ignore responses made by black students and may address the class as if no black students were present. Based on my research, black nursing students felt a great deal of discrimination throughout their collegiate program (Tucker-Allen, 1991). Hall and

Sandler (1982) state that faculty behaviors which may indicate lower expectations of minority students include ignoring, interrupting, maintaining physical distance, avoiding eye contact, offering little guidance and criticism, and attributing success to luck or factors other than ability. Minority women in higher education, therefore, face the effects of double stereotypes based on both gender and race.

BLACK WOMEN IN HIGHER EDUCATION

Gall (1990) indicates:

> In a tight budgetary climate, it is often acceptable to women to assume the duties of two jobs and receive compensation for only one with possibly a stipend for the other. Too often, women are placed in acting positions for one or two years, and then not considered seriously for the position that they handled adeptly. Are women more in jeopardy now than before? We cannot let these injustices continue but should publicly speak out and inform various professional organizations about the atrocities. The scenarios are obvious, but it is imperative that we develop solutions.
>
> Women of color bring a rich cultural heritage to the academy which provides enrichment to students, colleagues and the institution. (Our presence, in many ways, is the conscience of the institution.) We must endeavor to enlighten students about the contributions of ethnic groups and the significance of these contributions to their history. (p. 1)

Gall (1991) includes among the many factors that have impeded the progress of black women in higher education: inability to establish a good mentoring or nurturing affiliation with colleagues, ostracism, inability to identify key players of the inner circle, inability to share research with colleagues for possible feedback or collaboration, and inaccessibility to opportunities for funding or information on how to qualify for promotion.

Darlene Clark Hine (Pond, 1991), editor of the sixteen-volume series *Black Women in the United States History,* author of *Black Women in White,* a history of black women in the nursing profession, editor of *Eyes on the Prize,* and noted historian from Michigan State University, picked up Gall's theme when she stated in a recent interview that she views

> multicultural education as being a state of consciousness . . . how we go about the process of including with dignity and with elegance, the contributions of all people to the making of American society . . . it was wrong for us to teach for so long a dominant narrative that privileged elite white males essentially created this country. (p. 3)

Cook (1991) relates that just before her death, Barbara Deming, an early feminist, emphasized that the feminist movement will get nowhere until white women learn how to work with and understand women of color. She felt that white women faced a dual challenge, how to liberate themselves from patriarchal modes and also how to confront their long legacy of racism. White nursing faculty must understand their role in the interplay of minority relations both as viewed by minority students and female minority faculty members. They must also be cognizant of the views held by white male professors in the dominant university culture and how these views impact upon minority relations and longevity.

THE SEARCH FOR MINORITY FACULTY

Minority Students

Almost all universities and schools of nursing are searching for minority students and faculty members. The lack of progress in enrollment and graduation rates for minorities can be traced to the view held by some that quality and diversity are mutually exclusive. These persons believe that affirmative action and equal employment opportunity programs have allowed universities to hire more minority faculty who are less qualified than white faculty and that students who do not meet admission standards are being admitted. Faculty must confront these negative, untrue, and unsubstantiated views if they wish to correct past historical injustices and move into the 21st century.

The Study Group on Human Resources for Health (1989), part of the Association of Academic Health Centers, noted that:

> nursing schools should enhance student recruitment efforts aimed at minorities and nontraditional applicant pools, including men, and individuals who may be considering a second career or a return to the workforce. Recruitment efforts should be targeted not only at students in high school, but also at those in the junior high schools. (p. 5)

Two programs are outstanding in their effort to achieve these goals: the college of nursing at the University of Illinois at Chicago, funded by the Robert Wood Johnson Foundation and the school of nursing at Indiana University in Gary, Indiana, where students in the 11th grade take nursing courses while still in high school.

Roberts, Minnick, Ginzberg, and Curran (1989) argue that

> there is a major need to improve the recruiting of individuals from poor and minority backgrounds into nursing. Urban hospitals that serve the poor communities—and the nursing schools connected with them—have a special obligation and opportunity to provide career advancement to a cross section of the community they serve, while simultaneously doing something to meet their own staffing needs. (p. 19)

It has been found that minority students are more likely to succeed if there are minority faculty employed in the nursing program. How do you find minority nursing faculty?

Minority Faculty

Finding minority faculty has been almost an impossible task in the not too distant past. I would like to illustrate this point by briefly mentioning how and why I founded the Association of Black Nursing Faculty in Higher Education, Inc. (ABNF). With permission from my dissertation committee, I included two questions asking whether any minority faculty members were employed at the 18 schools of nursing included in my study. After graduation from Northwestern University, I then called the schools of nursing which indicated having minority faculty members and requested their names and addresses. I then invited all of them ($N=42$) to my home for a Saturday brunch (held on September 6, 1986). When the group met, 21 had responded, it was unanimous that we should meet again and that a formalized group should be formed. Ruby Steele, Sonia Baker, and I met in Springfield, Illinois, at the Days Inn and developed bylaws patterned after those of Sigma Theta Tau. On March 1, 1987, these bylaws were accepted by the founding group. Our first elections were held in May 1987, at Bradley University in Peoria, Illinois.

One of the primary goals of ABNF is to assist black nursing faculty members to meet tenure requirements, specifically research and publishing. We have encouraged our members to earn doctorates, to begin research projects, to develop fundable research proposals, to write and to publish. ABNF publishes both a quarterly newsletter and a quarterly journal which assists members in these efforts. Our membership has stabilized at 129, which is about 25 percent of all black nursing faculty teaching in baccalaureate and higher degree programs accredited by the National League for Nursing. We serve as a conduit for the recruitment of black nursing faculty for jobs located throughout the country and we are beginning to speak out both as a member of the Nursing Organization Liaison Forum (NOLF) and as concerned providers on health care issues as they relate to minorities.

RESEARCH RESULTS OF BLACK FACULTY AND STUDENTS

Ruby Steele, Sonia Baker, and I (1986) found that 96 percent of black nursing faculty teaching in baccalaureate and higher degree programs approximated national averages of 96 percent female and 4 percent male. The mean age of respondents was 40 years, with a standard deviation of 11.5 years. Forty-five percent of the respondents taught at schools of nursing in the southeast. Twenty percent taught at historically black colleges and universities and 80 percent at white institutions. Ninety-three percent worked full-time. These had worked at their present job for 7.9 mean years, with a standard deviation of 6.5. For these, the modal number of years was one and the median was six with over 50 percent working at their present job for six years or less. Almost 75 percent of those working full-time were either assistant or associate professors. Over one-third of them were tenured (44 percent at historically black colleges and universities and 33 percent at white institutions), with 14 percent at white institutions on the non-tenure track.

Our research results showed that black faculty members have not been fully integrated or socialized into the academic milieu of higher education as evidenced by the almost total lack of participation or inclusion in those scholarly activities which serve as a benchmark for academic success and professorial advancement. For example, black faculty members have not been awarded any fellowships, scholarships, or merit awards. They have written no books, chapters in books, or monographs. They have not published in either refereed or nonrefereed journals, have not published jointly, and have not been asked to publish jointly by their peers. They have attended professional conferences but have not presented papers at these conferences. They have not served as editor, board member, reviewer of manuscripts, or reviewer of research or grant proposals. They have also not been a member of a site review team.

Since it would seem that black faculty members are not being approached by their peers to publish jointly, black faculty members must actively seek out the collaboration of peers and others in conducting research and publishing. On the other hand, professional journals may be already receiving manuscripts from black faculty members concerning minority issues but these journals may not be accepting these manuscripts for publication. If this is the case, the profession needs to be apprised of this negative behavior and its consequences.

There also is an unequal distribution of black nursing faculty members by region, with almost half being employed in the southeast. It would seem that black faculty who are not tenured have nothing to lose by seeking employment in those regions with few to no black faculty. Our research also indicated that almost half of all black faculty members do not have any black advisees. Few black students, undergraduate as well as graduate, are being assigned to black faculty members as advisees.

SUMMARY

In this chapter, I attempted to explicate and highlight some of the interrelationships which exist in higher education between white male and female faculty members from a minority perspective. I discussed the effect of attitudes on the success of minority students and faculty in light of projected demographic changes. I hope that white female faculty members will become more cognizant of how negative attitudes impact upon both their own performance in higher education and also how the inculcation of these attitudes can be transferred to minority faculty members with devastating results. Change is difficult in all spheres of life, but without some modicum of change, life will go on as usual. Minority faculty members and students deserve at the very least a fair chance in the game we call higher education.

REFERENCES

American Association of Colleges of Nursing. (1991). *Relieving the nursing shortage among minorities.* Washington, DC: Author.

Big gain in nursing students lifts hopes amid a shortage. (1990, December 28). *The New York Times,* p. A1, 18.

Cook, B. W. (1991). *A review of black women in United States history.* Brooklyn: Carlson Publishing.

Gall, L. R. (1990, February). An endangered species: Black women in higher education. *The ABWHE Newsletter, 10*(2), 1.

Gall, L. R. (1991, June). Diversity? *The ABWHE Newsletter, 11*(3), 1.

Hall, R. M., & Sandler, B. R. (1982). *The classroom climate: A chilly one for women?* Washington, DC: Association of American Colleges.

Pond, W. (1991, February 10). [Interview with Darlene Clark Hine]. *Soundings,* p. 1–4.

Roberts, M., Minnick, A., Ginsberg, E., & Curran, C. (1989). *A commonwealth fund paper: What to do about the nursing shortage.* New York: Commonwealth Fund.

Study Group on Human Resources for Health. (1989). *The supply and education of nurses.* (Policy Paper No. 1). Washington, DC: Association of Academic Health Centers.

Tucker-Allen, S., Steele, R., & Baker, S. (1990). A descriptive survey of black nursing faculty. *The ABNF Journal, 1*(1), 14–17.

Tucker-Allen, S., Steele, R., & Baker, S. (1988). *The mentoring role of black nursing faculty.* Unpublished manuscript.

Tucker-Allen, S. (1991). Minority student nurses' perceptions of their educational program. *The ABNF Journal, 2*(3), 50–63.

5

Educational Implications of Nursing Faculty Diversity

Ruby L. Steele

Current predictions regarding future health care needs refer to a global community which by the year 2000 will be a majority of minorities. The United States is rapidly becoming the most ethnically and culturally diverse society in the world. With that in view, nursing faculty as well as other health professionals must commit to preparing clinicians who can deliver culturally relevant care.

For purposes of discussion, minority denotes a perspective or position not held by the dominant culture. It does not necessarily mean greater population. American health care generally follows the western biomedical model. Although recently there have been movements toward holistic perspectives and some eastern concepts, basically, the germ theory and doctrine of specific etiology prevail. The World Health Organization in the Declaration of Alma-Ata (1978) proposed a model for primary health care for all by 2000. Some have seen this as an area of concern for nursing educators. Graduates of today need to know assessment procedures from a multicultural perspective that extends beyond the confines of their personal cultural view.

A global community that should be of the most concern at the moment is the culturally diverse United States community. In communities, industry, schools, and health care institutions, there are people of many nationalities, ethnicities, and cultures. Much of the national success is a tribute to what is referred to as the American cultural characteristic of tolerance, based on rational pragmatism.

Many schools of nursing provide opportunity for students to study abroad as part of the curriculum. The majority of students, however, do not have this experience for reasons of access, availability, finances, or personal circumstances. Whether students are the fortunate few to study in another country or not, they will encounter culturally diverse clientele in whatever clinical area they practice.

DIVERSE CULTURES

Professions, nations, institutions, and corporations, like people, have cultures. The same principles of patterned responses, values transmission, and shared norms apply. Change occurs constantly, although it may be barely perceptible at times. Like the clothes we wear, culture is part of our cover and identification. It can be modified when necessary without total change or abandonment of the basic structure. Certain cultural standards provide security and guidelines that help to mediate between the social milieu and individual personality. Culture shapes our perception of reality and influences the form that conflict takes. It also defines what we call deviance and how we deal with it.

In nursing, a main effect of the split between service and education has been the emergence of two subcultures. Despite basic common values, education and service have developed along somewhat parallel lines. Some hold that nurses in the service sector enjoy more comfort and security than those in academic settings. Granted, we are newer to higher education than to the practice area. Theory building and academic progress requires different competencies than those acquired through the application of practice models. For some, there is a great need to catch up, keep pace, and hold our own in the ever elusive quest for truth. The road to tenure is not the same as the one to clinical competence, and certainly not an easier one. Recruiting and retaining faculty that are culturally diverse means that academic institutions will have to actively seek out and support candidates that need and deserve such support.

CHANGING FACES

Demographics for both nursing faculty and students have changed tremendously during the last 40 years. Earlier students were generally white, female, unmarried, and from rural and working class backgrounds. Scholarly inquiry was not emphasized nor did the rigorous training allow for much reflection or discovery. Teaching responsibility fell to the head nurse and the physicians. The model was one of apprenticeship and on-the-job training.

After World War II, societal forces converged to change nursing and nursing education dramatically. Responding to the nursing shortage, federal loans and grants opened the way for the disadvantaged and culturally diverse. How well nursing has responded to the changes is an open question and certainly a fair one. Men are no longer a rarity and older students above high school graduation age are commonplace. Members of minority groups have entered in greater numbers since nursing education became available and accessible via community colleges. It is a profession that is almost recession proof. Indeed, many people who today study nursing have a prior degree. What we see today is a much more heterogeneous student population that reflects the larger society to a great degree.

ASSESSMENT

As a result of these changes, the student population is more diverse. The clientele is also more diverse. We can predict with a high degree of certainty that students today cannot expect to work only with clients who resemble them culturally and ethnically. Nevertheless, faculty is less diverse. Consequently, the educational environment for students is not as reflective of society as it might be.

Some institutions have taken steps to address this mismatch via innovative recruiting and marketing strategies, fellowships, teacher exchanges, and adjunct appointments. There appears to be consensus that when taught by faculty of other cultural or ethnic groups students benefit greatly. Still, there remain schools of nursing that have no minority faculty at all. Data from student responses and evaluations have indicated positive outcomes; culturally diverse interaction should precede any community health nursing practicum. Encounters, in my own experience with multicultural faculty, have positive outcomes such as increased cultural awareness and sensitivity.

In a recent survey of students in a BSN completion program, there was a significant increase in posttest cultural awareness scores after students were taught transcultural content. One group came from small town settings and another from the inner city. A group of registered nurses, who did not take the course, served as control. It would be ideal, of course, if nursing education could be conducted in an environment that represented a diversity of perspectives and approaches. Such an atmosphere could speak volumes about respect and caring for the needs of all clients.

As educators our goals can be:

1. To provide resource faculty with curricula and support services necessary to implement procedures and policies that will prepare clinicians for service to a multicultural clientele.

2. To increase faculty diversity by institutional commitment, evidenced by creative marketing strategies and use of network resources when vacancies occur.

3. To promote cultural awareness through statements in the conceptual framework and content mapping, and through ongoing assessment for transcultural concepts in the curriculum.
4. To monitor curricula for consistency and integration across courses.
5. To provide ongoing faculty development through the use of consultants and to provide sensitivity workshops that encourage and support collegiality.
6. To assess the environment to determine whether minority faculty perceive it to be hospitable, indifferent, or hostile.

REFERENCES

Atwell, R. (1988, January). Minority participation in higher education: We need a new momentum. Paper presented at the annual meeting of the American Council on Education, Washington, DC.

Cooper, R., & Smith, B. (1990, October). Achieving a diverse faculty. *American Association Higher Education, Bulletin*, 10–11.

Curtin, L. (1990). Creating a culture of competence. Editorial in *Nursing Management*, 21(9), 7–8.

DeSantis, L. (1988). The relevance of transcultural to international nursing. *International Nursing Review, 35,* 110.

Elder, O. (1990). Looking to the 21st century in schools of allied health. *Journal of Allied Health, 19,* 30.

Hegyvary, S. (1990). Education: A new melting pot. *Journal of Professional Nursing,* 6(3), 135.

Mercer, J. (1991). Faculty diversity: A strength of historically black colleges and universities scholars say. *Black Issues in Higher Education,* 8(6), 6–5.

6

Valuing Cultural Diversity in Nursing Faculty

Joanette Pete McGadney

*M*anaging and valuing cultural diversity are becoming the corporate watchwords of the decade, not because corporations are becoming kinder and gentler toward minority groups, but because corporations want to survive. One compelling challege results from a drastically changing workforce. White, native-born men are no longer a hegemonic majority in the United States workplace, and this change will be even more stark around the year 2000.

Most employers and managers are not prepared to deal with cultural diversity. In fact, many grew up having little contact with other cultures. Employers and managers are actually culturally deprived; their graduate school text books did not cover the kinds of situations that arise in today's multicultural settings. But, some organizations are taking aggressive steps to meet the demographic challenge of the 1990s by establishing such positions as director of valuing differences or director of multicultural planning and design.

Historically, nurses have recognized that the United States is a salad bowl of individuals from various ethnic and cultural backgrounds. Nurses have long been forced into an awareness that people are indeed different and that, because of these differences, patients respond to health and illness in culturally specific ways. Today, most nursing curricula include multicultural concepts, racial and cultural models, and transcultural philosophies. Therefore, students participate in cultural diversity training that focuses on self-awareness, ethnicity, and knowledge of culture and its functions. They learn to recognize and overcome cultural barriers to the delivery of health care. Their practice is designed to address certain predetermined cultural and ehtnic needs of different groups within our society. Faculty also make specific efforts to recruit and retain students from different ethnic, gender, and cultural backgrounds.

Still, nursing faculty have not focused as much attention on recruiting, maintaining, or valuing diversity among its faculty. For the most part, nursing faculty resemble corporate United States in that most of the nursing faculty are white. Ironically, the literature points out there are many benefits to having and valuing a diverse nursing faculty. These benefits derive from the ability to recruit the best talent from entire labor pools. So, one can expect greater creativity and innovation, a broader range of skills, better decisions based on different perspectives, and better service to diverse patients and clients.

Maintaining and valuing a diverse faculty facilitates a broader, more enlightened approach to health care delivery. A diverse faculty is able to help students eliminate some of the culturally inaccurate and inappropriate judgements that often lead to ineffective and unsafe nursing care. In addition, a diverse faculty is desirable because of their interaction with clients.

One author has developed a framework to explore the complexities and depth of cultural diversity (Figure 1). By examining two basic dimensions, the researcher can explore the challenges that come from attempting to understand and value cultural diversity. This two-dimensional framework is a cognitive guide for locating and working through the challenge. The two dimensions are: (1) breadth of awareness of the complexity of the issues, and (2) depth of understanding or insight.

The horizontal axis describes the breadth of awareness. Individuals must comprehend the complexity of issues based on their personal experience in an organization and move from there to the

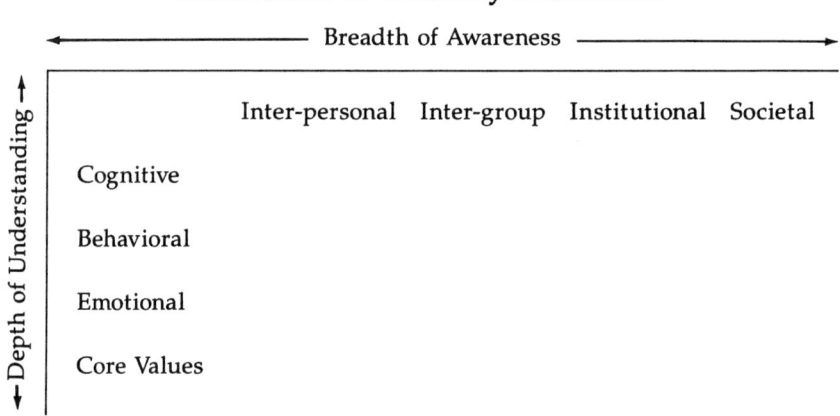

Figure 1
Dimensions of Diversity Framework

←——————— Breadth of Awareness ———————→

	Inter-personal	Inter-group	Institutional	Societal
Cognitive				
Behavioral				
Emotional				
Core Values				

↑↓ Depth of Understanding

group, institution, and society's comprehension of the issues. The vertical axis depicts the depth of understanding as the range of responses individuals have about the issues. Comprehension of the issues proceed from the cognitive to the behavioral to the emotional and to the core value levels of understanding. Movement along this dimension indicates the individual's thinking, feelings, actions, and fundamental values.

While the framework can be assessed for its simplicity, it can also be employed as a guide for diagnosing or intervening in implementing a program to value cultural diversity among nursing faculty. The major benefit of the framework becomes obvious when group members give life to the model by using it to facilitate their own exploration of the complexities of valuing diversity. By using this framework, faculty would learn that other faculty have different personal experiences, awareness of group identity, and knowledge about institutional and societal conditions. Faculty would realize that each member of the group brings an enormous range of ideas, feelings, behaviors, and values. Managing and valuing diversity requires understanding the two core dimensions of the framework. Valuing diversity will not evolve along a straight path. Nevertheless, the realization will grow that the best way for people to work effectively is to recognize and celebrate each other's differences. The process to value diversity includes several key steps:

1. *Stripping away stereotypes:* Stereotypes are powerful and effective. They prevent a change in opinion about people who belong within the stereotyped group. A stereotype is an exaggerated belief associated with a category. Its function is to justify conduct in relation to that category. Stereotypes hurt individuals particularly when based on invalid conclusions and when those conclusions remain untested and unchanged. Learning about differences is the best way to eliminate stereotypes.

2. *Learning to listen and to probe for the differences in people's assumptions:* Often when erroneous assumptions are made about a different cultural group, no attempt has been made to analyze the assumptions.

3. *Building authentic and significant relationships with people one regards as different:* Even though many recognize cultural differences, the perception of the differences is viewed as a deviation from the norm, that is, the norm being set by white, middle-class United States. What is needed is acceptance of culturally different behaviors as a unique part of the individual's human experience. Using a diversity framework, developing an understanding of the process involved in the management of diversity, is not going to automatically guarantee success with a

group of nursing faculty. Obstacles will rise. For example, a group may have unwritten rules for success, reflected in attitudes about what is important, how the organization does its work, how employees are to behave, and how they are to be rewarded. In this case, what is written may differ greatly from what is practiced and it may never occur to the group members that someone, particularly one who has a different background, may not be aware of the unwritten rules.

4. *Exclusion from the club:* Relationships are central to an achievement and being a member of the *club* may be as important as hard work and competence. Exclusion from the *club* prevents members of the minority group from being well known by other *club* members and, thus, minority members are less likely to be promoted.

5. *Untested assumptions:* People from different cultural groups behave differently and that difference affects their relationship to the organization. People from one ethnic group are not inherently better or worse than those from another group; they are simply different. It is judgment, not recognition, of cultural differences that leads to inappropriate, racist, sexist, homophobic, and ethnocentric attitudes and behavor.

6. *Real cultural differences:* Cultures are different. What motivates one worker might completely inhibit another. Cultural differences affect the values people bring to the workplace. Different people feel differently about their roles in an organization, the contribution they can make, and how they want to be recognized for their efforts.

The successful nursing faculty must be able to build work environments that accommodate diverse groups comfortably. It must be able to capitalize on the groups' differences because they are strengths. Our challenge is not only to accommodate diversity, but to actually use it to bring new and richer perspectives to nursing education, to clients, and to the whole social climate.

Whereas valuing diversity is an established mode of operation in some companies, it is not practiced in others. Even the most progressive organization may have offices or divisions in regions of the country where more work needs to be done. Nursing faculty is no exception. Plenty of companies and universities have given lip service to the idea of managing a diverse workforce. Nevertheless, they end up with few changes because they have failed to establish accountability. Just as with corporate United States, if nursing is to survive in the 21st century, faculty diversity is a must.

REFERENCES

Adams, L. A., & Nelson, P. B. (1990). Multiculturalism: Its challenges to nursing. *The UT Nurse News Journal*, 4–5.

Adler, N. J. (1986). Cultural syngergy: Managing the impact of cultural diversity. *The 1986 annual: Developing human resources*, 229–238.

Copeland, L. (1990). Learning to manage a multicultural workforce. *Training*, 52–56.

Edwards, A. (1991, January). Cultural diversity in today's corporation: The enlightened manager. *Working Woman*, 45–62.

Glynn, N. (1986). Multiculturalism in nursing: Implications for faculty development. *Journal of Nursing Education, 25*(1), 39–41.

Kirkham, K. (1990). Dimensions of diversity: A basic framework. *Journal of Counseling and Development, 69*(1), 21–26.

Loden, M., & Loeser, R. H. (1991). Working diversity: Managing the differences. *The Bureaucrat-The Journal for Public Managers*, Spring, 21.

Mandell, B., & Kohler-Gray, S. (1990). Management development that values diversity. *Personnel*, 41–47.

Thomas, R. R. (1990). From affirmative action to affirming diversity. *Harvard Business Review*, 107–117.

Tuck, I. (1984). Strategies for integrating African-American culture into transcultural nursing. *Journal of Nursing Education, 23*(6), 261–262.

7

Nursing from the International Perspective

Jeanette Lancaster

*T*here are a multitude of issues that could be covered under the topic nursing from the international perspective. I have chosen to focus on four: (1) Is it appropriate for an affluent country, like the United States, in the midst of a nursing shortage to actively recruit foreign nurse graduates from less affluent countries? (2) Is it the role of a highly developed country to assist lesser-developed countries in educating their nurses so that the latter can make a difference in the quality of nursing care and education at home? (3) How important is it for nursing curricula to provide students with content and experiences in international health care? (4) What can be the role of a philanthropic foundation whose mission is to improve the quality of nursing, medicine, and public health in selected Asian countries?

RECRUITMENT OF FOREIGN NURSE GRADUATES: RIGHT OR WRONG?

Dvorak and Waymack (1991) conclude, after analyzing the recruitment of foreign nurses, that there is nothing unethical about such practice. Nevertheless they are not convinced that recruiting foreign nurses is the best way to solve the nursing shortage in the United States. Because "in all countries, nurses constitute one of the most important health care delivery resources" (p. 120), country officials view recruitment of their nurses as a drain of a vital national resource. In my visits to Kenya, Thailand, and China, I have found that health care officials are suspicious of the United States because of our reputation for facilitating brain drain from their countries. Recruitment of foreign nurses is big business (Glittenburg, 1989). Particularly, English-speaking countries are easy targets for head hunters. In recent years, heavy recruitment has spread to Nepal, Pakistan, the Dominican Republic, Jamaica, China, Haiti, Guyana, India, South Korea, Columbia, and Ecuador.

According to Glittenburg (1989) there are three main concerns that must be acknowledged regarding the recruitment of foreign nurse graduates:

1. Exploitation of the graduating nurse
2. Depletion of the nursing supply in the foreign country
3. Licensure of foreign nurses in the United States without adequate clinical preparation.

Exploitation occurs when short-term solutions, such as the importation of nurses, replaces addressing long-range reasons for a nursing shortage in the first place. One can say that depletion is simply not right. For example, the Philippines has one of the lowest health status indexes of any country in the World Health Organization's Western Pacific Region, yet it exports tremendous numbers of nurses to the United States (Glittenburg, 1989). Ortin (1990) gives vivid examples of the effects of the nurse migration from her country. The Philippines Nursing Association estimates that 96,900 nurses are needed in their country. Hospitals have annual turnover rates ranging from 5 to 59 percent. Migration of nurses leads to the following problems for those who stay:

1. Heavier workloads
2. Unnecessary overtime
3. Burnout
4. Absenteeism
5. Job dissatisfaction.

In countries that experience considerable nurse migration, schools of nursing come to be run by people who do not always meet set standards. Despite a lack of faculty with graduate degrees to serve as administrators and teachers, more schools are opening. Political pressure to produce more nurses for export is so great that the production of nurses for export supersedes the country's need to retain the nurses it educates.

LICENSURE ISSUES

Particularly, licensure has been a difficult problem. The United States has a carefully monitored regulatory system with strict standards for the level of clinical preparation in undergraduate nursing programs. It has been accepted that graduates who pass the United States' licensure exams have a minimal, yet expected, level of clinical competency. On the other hand, there is no way to verify the level of clinical competence of foreign nurse graduates coming from countries that do not require a licensure examination.

During past nursing shortages, when agencies scoured the world looking for nurses, many foreign nurses were misled about the circumstances surrounding their migration. Specifically, large numbers of foreign-educated nurses arrived in the United States only to discover that they were unable to pass the licensure exam. Between 1969 and 1978, more than 82,000 foreign nurse graduates immigrated to the United States; some 70,000 or 85 percent failed the licensure exam which tested for English language competency and knowledge of United States nursing practice. Unable to obtain an RN license, thousands of foreign nurses had to return home (Maroun and Serota, 1988).

Those who remained in the United States often suffered employment exploitation. They were relegated to low-paying assistant level jobs. Others practiced nursing illegally. This chaotic situation led the United States Immigration and Naturalization Service to ask the Division of Nursing within DHEW for assistance. At this time the Division of Nursing, the American Nurses' Association, and the National League for Nursing collaboratively established the Commission on Graduates of Foreign Nursing Schools (CGFNS) in 1977.

COMMISSION ON GRADUATES OF FOREIGN NURSING SCHOOLS

CGFNS, an independent, private, nonprofit organization has a twofold mission (Maroun & Serota, 1988):

- To identify foreign nurse graduates who would be likely to pass the RN licensure exam
- To insure high quality nursing care for the American public.

CGFNS carefully assesses applicants to determine if the quality of their nursing education meets minimal standards and includes content in all clinical areas. The exam is offered twice a year in 43 cities around the world. Over the past decade, CGFNS has identified nearly 56,000 nurses who were eligible to take its qualifying examination; of these, over 25,000 have passed the exam and 89 percent or 23,000 went on to pass the RN licensure exam.

ENCOURAGING A GLOBAL PERSPECTIVE

There is increasing interest in foreign nurses coming to the United States to study so they can then assume leadership positions in either nursing education or administration in their home countries. In the 1960s and 1970s, the education of nurses from other countries was promoted and sponsored by agencies such as USAID, WHO, UNESCO, and Project Hope. In the 1980s, and now into the 1990s, the financing shifted to foreign governments, private foundations, and church organizations (Mooneyhan, 1986).

Many will argue that it is the role of an affluent country, enriched by a large cadre of well-educated nurses, to assist other countries and other nurses to improve their educational levels. This role may not include the actual giving of money or provision of free tuition, but may be in the form of gifts in kind or extra assistance to students.

As the boundaries of the world come closer and as the barriers to collaboration break down, it is of vital importance that students have opportunities to learn about health care in countries other than their own. Perhaps the best way to learn this is to travel to another country and participate, even briefly, in a nursing experience with health care providers. When travel to another country is not possible, the second best option is to have students from other countries join your student body and share their own values, education, and experience. The third option is to integrate content into the curriculum that emphasizes other cultures. With so many nurses available who have worked, lived, studied, and traveled to other countries, this is no longer difficult.

ONE FOUNDATION'S APPROACH TO CHANGING THE EDUCATIONAL LEVEL OF NURSING: CHINA MEDICAL BOARD PROGRAM

Soon after becoming President of the China Medical Board in 1987, Dr. Bill Sawyer established the Committee on Graduate Nursing Education (COGNE). I became chair of this six-person committee. In 1988, we began developing a program to bring nurses from the People's Republic of China (PRC) to the United States to earn master's degrees. These Chinese students could then go back and become the faculty for the eight new BSN programs that began in 1985.

From 1951 until 1985 there was no baccalaureate nursing education in the PRC. During the twelve years of the Cultural Revolution period, there was no nursing education at all. This means that nurses educated in Chinese colleges are either very old or quite young. These nurses are developing the same tensions that have been present in the United States in the past: very capable diploma nurses versus new, young BSN graduates.

Our program set out to finance and admit 16 Chinese nurses to the six schools represented by members of COGNE. Participating COGNE schools were chosen based on a willingness to take risks and, if needed, to bend policies to accomplish the goal of admitting the Chinese students. For example, entering students did not have baccalaureate degrees. The President of each participating Chinese University was asked to choose the two most capable nurses on the faculty and to certify in writing that they had the equivalent of a United States baccalaureate degree. The students had to satisfactorily pass both the Test of English as a Foreign Language (TOEFL) and the Graduate Record Examination (GRE). They also had to be willing to leave their families for two years. Sixteen students were chosen.

In his travels through Asia, Dr. Sawyer was able to talk with almost all applicants and could attest to their ability to speak and understand English. During the summer of 1990, two COGNE members with limited experience with international students accompanied Dr. Sawyer to China to learn more about Chinese education, health care, and conventions. The Chinese students, on the other hand, were scheduled to begin an intensive orientation and acculturation program at the University of Tennessee from early June 1990 until mid-August. Only five of the 16 arrived in the United States in time to participate in the summer program. Fifteen arrived by August and one was unable to get the necessary papers processed prior to the start of the school year. Partially, reasons for the delay seemed to lie with the American universities, which had established appropriate deadlines for a June rather than an August entry into the United States. Also, the layers of paperwork that had to be done for passports, visas, and other exit papers was enormous. We learned that we needed to start earlier.

The students have done remarkably well in their academic work. They are dedicated to their studies; they compete well with American students; they have a good mastery of the language; they have a good nursing education. The only exception is in psychosocial areas. They do have difficulty participating actively in class, because they are not accustomed to the give and take that characterizes American classrooms. They are particularly strong in science courses. They do not find pathophysiology and physical assessment overly difficult. A factor limiting their advanced learning, however, is that some states restrict their clinical practice even under faculty supervision.

The program to bring Chinese students to learn nursing under the COGNE's supervision has taught us that:

1. Chinese students are very resourceful.

2. They immediately find and are found by local Chinese communities.

3. Some students have suffered hardships due to leaving husbands and small children in China. Still, they speak dispassionately about hardships.

4. Older students (30 years and older) remember the Cultural Revolution. Many come from educated families directly affected by the Cultural Revolution. Hence, the freedom found in America is unusual for them.

5. Because there is concern that some students will try to immigrate permanently, thereby defeating the purpose of the program, we will wait at least one year following program completion by the current students before restarting the cycle. This will assure us that students go home and perform effectively in their new roles.

REFERENCES

Glittenburg, J. E. (1989). Foreign nurse recruitment: Conflicts and concerns. *Journal of Professional Nursing, 5*(6), 303, 353.

Maroun, V. M., & Serota, C. (1988). Demanding quality when foreign nurses are in demand. *Nursing & Health Care, 9*(7), 361–363.

McQuaid, E., & Waymack, M. H. (1991). Is it ethical to recruit foreign nurses? *Nursing Outlook, 39*(3), 120–123.

Mooney, E. L. (1986). International dimensions of nursing and health care in baccalaureate and higher degree nursing programs in the United States. *Journal of Professional Nursing, 2*(2), 82–90.

Ortin, E. L. (1990). The brain drain as viewed by an exporting country. *International Nursing Review, 37*(5), 340–344.

PART FOUR

Nursing and the Community

8

A Community-Based Health Program for the Homeless

Tim Porter-O'Grady and Lorine Spencer

During the past decade, the economic changes in America have resulted in many changes for society. Constraining economic circumstances have resulted in a considerable change of consciousness for most Americans. Since the founding of the nation, it has been the land of opportunity and unlimited resources. It has only been during the Great Depression and the 1970s that the nation has become aware that resources are not unlimited and that constraint is a fact of economic and social life. Unable to incorporate that reality into the American culture, the nation has been driven into further constraint by a negative balance of trade and the accumulation of an extensive debt (Beatty, 1990).

In order to adjust and compensate for decreasing sources of funding, Congress has been reducing the number of dollars allocated to a whole range of public-sponsored programs. In order to survive, programs have had to look at alternative mechanisms for assuring that those they serve are cared for in ways that more effectively use diminished resources. Programs have adjusted their service characteristics and parameters and even tightened up their criteria for furnishing services. As a result of the constraining economic circumstances, however, even greater demand has been placed on human service providers. A diminished economy creates an increasing demand on social and human services already affected by the same economic downturn. Thus emerges a cycle of diminishing supply and increasing demand with all the burdens on the service provider that implies (Lamm, 1991).

One of the major outcomes of constraining economic circumstances has been an increase in the numbers of Americans who have become dispossessed and are left homeless. Atlanta, because of its southern climate and social circumstances has had more than its share of homeless persons. While Atlanta is not unique in the fact that it has a large homeless population, it is unique in its response to the homeless. Like all large cities in America, Atlanta has a homeless population that is very visible.

It is estimated by the Atlanta Task Force for the Homeless that there are up to 15,000 homeless persons in Atlanta, most of them residing in the central and inner city. During the winter months, the city shelters and the private sector sheltering community find it impossible to house the number of homeless seeking shelter. Many homeless persons remain outside of the sheltering support system, exposed to the elements.

Demands on the human services and health care system in the city of Atlanta become quickly overwhelmed by the increasing service load that homelessness provokes. Not only do the homeless swell the ranks of those who have no other service options, but they also bring unique health problems potentiated by exposure to the elements.

In the winter of 1986, a number of local health professionals began a private effort to bring some semblance of health care services to the homeless in the shelters. It soon became apparent, however, that their "tackle box" approach to health services was inadequate to the demand and that a more systematic approach would be required. Resources were slim and community interest was low, including interest from the health care system.

Because of the breadth of the problem, several nurse members of the volunteer group decided to undertake a concerted effort to address the health needs of the homeless by putting together a proposal for directed services to the homeless community and sheltered population. A proposal to a private foundation yielded a small grant that allowed for the purchase of a van and its outfitting with basic health equipment. A major volunteer program was constructed and a service schedule developed. A team of nurses, physicians, and other health professionals made regular and continuous visits to shelters, first, during the winter season and eventually for the full year.

Volunteer service was a great contribution to the health needs of the homeless but it soon became apparent that following homeless persons and assuring continuity of care was compromised by the logistics of a voluntary program. The sponsors and providers of the volunteer services decided to create a continuous and full time consortium of service providers and to construct a nurse-managed program for service delivery for the homeless.

Working with the Task Force for the Homeless and the United States Public Health Service, a federal grant was constructed and accepted for funding under the McKinney Homeless Assistance Act. With both the public and private funding, the nurse-managed health service community project for homeless health care was initiated.

A Community-Based Health Program for the Homeless 63

Called the Atlanta Community Health Program (ACHP), it formed a coalition of partners in both the public and private sector to assure a multi–level of health and social services so that the full range of service needs of the homeless could be addressed.

The program grew from "tackle boxes" and a single van to four mobile units, two fixed clinic sites, one for women and children and the other for men, and a major diagnostic mobile unit for special examination and lab testing. Nurse practitioners, assistive health advocates, and various social service support persons make regular visits to one of the 26 shelter clinics or wherever else they are needed to find and identify homeless persons with health needs. These nurses and health professionals also follow up with clients already seen but needing further attention. Through use of a computerized database, the nurses can track and follow clients and identify their health needs and history wherever they may find them. Through use of physician affiliations, an employed physician, and clinical protocols, additional health services can be provided and referrals can be made to other services and health settings.

During the first year of operation, the program experienced 6,747 visits. In the fourth year of service, that number doubled to 12,647 visits. This indicated a growing use of the clinical services and a growing demand for the health services they provided. As the number of uninsured and indigent continues to increase in the area, it is expected that the demand for these health services will continue to grow. During the first year, support for the nurse-run program was tenuous with some fear regarding whether nurses could meet the demand and provide high level primary services. In the subsequent years, the nurses' credibility has grown dramatically and relationships between the hospital and health care community with the homeless health program has grown significantly.

As those with substance abuse problems and persons with AIDS increase in the community, the demands on the health services of the ACHP and its health teams will accelerate. Anticipating this increase in use, the nursing leadership has worked diligently to form coalitions with the state and county services to connect and expand services for substance abuse and persons with AIDS. These coalitions lead to the provision of newer services on site, such as HIV testing and counselling and substance abuse services.

The model of bringing health services to the client, within the person's environment, and creating a mobile context to health care services, is unique to the nursing role. Linking those in need to the continuum of health services that can address needs where they arise is vital. Health care focus can more frequently be on prevention as well as treatment where necessary. The ACHP shows what nurses are capable of accomplishing and how newer models of health care can be both efficient and cost effective.

BUILDING HEALTH COALITIONS

As health care becomes more complex and more expensive, services directed to those on the periphery of society become affected by the economic and resource constraints that budget priorities create. The shrinking availability of dollars forces service providers to look at what they are doing and how they are providing services. Duplication of services and unilateral program structures can no longer survive the shrinking economic base of those programs directed to underserved people. Effective use of dollars and construction of services call for a radical redesign of the structure of service programs and relationships if appropriate levels and kinds of services needed are to survive and continue to meet the needs for which they were designed.

Effective program structures call for a new approach to service relationships and program design. Free-standing and unilateral service structures that are self-defined and self-supported are no longer viable or even effective as a way of arraying services. There are neither the dollars nor the human resources sufficient for such programs. The need to interface programs and services, to create a complex of relationships in service provision, surfaces as the only viable mechanism for comprehensive service frameworks and program survival. As a reflection of this reality, the ACHP was designed and constructed as a service coalition (Porter-O'Grady, Patti, & McDonagh, 1990).

Forming coalitions is no easy task. A number of behaviors moderate against their initial success:

- Preexisting service structures that were well designed and operating in place successfully when funding was adequate
- Poor link with other similar or related service programs, which provides no urge for communication
- Strong competition between existing or emerging programs for available or new funds
- A strong segmentation of the population served into categories of service that often did not encourage a systems approach to meeting human needs (e.g., social programs, food programs, mental health programs, physical health programs)
- A structural design that expected program clients to come to the service provider at a time when the clients' ability to access the provider was severely compromised
- The inability of some programs to establish a level of credibility in delivering the services promised

- Costs of individual programs not justified by the breadth or depth of services actually provided.

The growth of an intensive service bureaucracy, coming under the heading of a number of different program identifiers at both the state and federal levels, simply exacerbated the differentiation and lack of connection between like and supporting service structures. The costs and human resource demands of supporting the administrative configuration alone mitigate against an affordable and cost effective framework for service provision to the underserved. This is especially true in today's economic environment. Clearly, a major retooling of the service framework is in order.

Building service coalitions inherently comes up against traditional service structures. Such building demands that the parties look at their services within the context of the range of services provided as a collective. Driving the circumstances which point to service coalitions are the limited resources available and the need for a more effective manner for delivering services. Common ground must be sought out and relationships negotiated both to the extent of the need and the nature of the services provided.

Integration becomes an additional value that emerges in collaborative or collective relationship. The ability to provide a composite of services which deals with the related needs of those served becomes a cornerstone of the collaborated relationship. Somehow, a mosaic of services has to be provided in ways that can benefit the persons served but also services have to relate one to the other so that a benefit is achieved and some valid outcome or change is produced. In this scenario, the nature of the relationship and the character of the service must be worked out at the outset. Each of the parties must be aware of their unique contribution and value that of the other members of the coalition. Successful initiation of service coalitions will depend to a great extent on the following:

- Common interest in service provision and relationship building

- Clearly defined grantee or program director established so that competition for the role is reduced

- Ability to connect services in a way that is mutually supportive and able to be integrated

- Ability to formalize specified service structures so that the appropriate service can meet the needs of a designated segment of the underserved

- Willingness to undertake the work of grant writing and document generation as expected

- Desire to extend the sharing of responsibility throughout the service system
- Comfort with collaboration and information sharing including the ability to adjust roles and functions to better facilitate the service relationships
- Willingness to take direction from the grantee or program or coalition coordinator. Ability to allow service providers to be responsible to others in the program coalition
- Flexibility to change service structures and functions to fit the needs of the population served.

Relationship building is a challenging process for all the parties. Since it is generally a new experience for many of the providers, the initial attempts at connection may require some political finesse. Often, the parties may not have ever connected with each other and, in some cases, may have even been competitors for scarce resources in the past. Some sensitivity to this reality can help the grantee in planning some of the initial activities in establishing a service relationship. Some helpful considerations are:

- An informal meeting of the parties at the outset, designed to introduce each to the other and to explore the character and content of the service coalition, is an important beginning.
- Presentation of a vision of the program introduced and coordinated by the grantee helps put form to the notions each brings to the relationship.
- Staying away from hard and fast rules in the beginning regarding the service concept prevents the formation of polarized positions and reactive attitudes that may create problems later on.
- Setting out time frames and role commitments in the proposal process helps give form to the effort and creates a purpose and direction for the participants in the beginning of the process.
- Using a facilitation technique for dialogue and concept exploration gets both presets and expectations on the table; it also helps to clarify and move the parties to stronger concerns regarding the proposed coalition and program.

The quality of the initial connections often sets the context for future relationships. An honest but respectful interaction can provide the baseline for the negotiation of roles over the life of the relationship. The program or coalition coordinator will need to recognize the political impact of coalition formation. Attention to the relationship along the continuum of program development and service delivery can assure successful interaction. Political processes will play a key role in the success of the enterprise. Underestimation of the relationship of external and internal alliances and their dynamic nature is frequently the source of greatest conflict and can cause the collapse of the coalition. Special attention must be paid to the following elements of relationship building:

- Each agency has internal constraints and possibilities. These must be understood and incorporated into the plan.

- Always, there are key players in each service agency who are not the same as those involved in planning. These key players may not be visible to the planners either. Key players must be acknowledged and incorporated into the relationship to the extent they affect it.

- Often, there are key leadership persons who are not a part of the coalition but who affect it. These persons must also be taken into consideration according to their influence or role.

- Communication must be continuous and sensitive to the needs of the parties. Each party will require different levels and kinds of communication. Program or coalition coordinators will have to individualize communication to each of the involved parties.

- In some circumstances, some members of the coalition may have some difficulty with other members or personality difficulties may arise. The program or coalition coordinator will have to make judgments regarding the appropriate approach in dealing with these members. Whenever possible, problem-solving strategies can be helpful. At other times the linkage may have to be provided by others in the coalition as necessary.

- Flexibility at the design stage of the coalition will pay off later on during the implementation phase. All members will have to recognize that there are many alterations in the proposal and implementation of the coalition driven by the vagaries of public policy, fiscal constraints, and modifications. Patience and good communication skills are a must for program or coalition coordinators in representing these realities to the participants.

Perhaps the most important of the above factors is that which relates to the political process. The one reality that emerges in any venture, specifically, human services, is the significance of relationships and their impact on the venture. All processes require the ability to make connections that facilitate their success. That cannot be done unilaterally or without involving and investing others in the effort. The more that reality is applied in program and service development, the greater the possibility of success in the venture.

Much of public politics has been directed to turf fighting and maintaining programmatic control. The psychology of that experience does not translate easily to service coalitions where the boundaries are less definitive and all relationships are subject to dialogue and negotiation. Some preparation for the change in behavior and relationship could be very helpful in expediting the coalition building process. Some of the constraints that may affect successful coalitions can often be addressed in the developmental process including strategies for problem resolution.

SOME CONSIDERATIONS REGARDING FUNDING

There is nothing as rife with political content as seeking support funding for the continued operation of a public, community-based program. This is of special consideration today when resources are scarce, regardless of the value of the work.

It is precisely because of this reality that funding planning becomes so important to the leadership of such programs. There are no major purveyors of funds breaking down the doors of service providers and looking to spend their money. There are a lot of valuable services competing heavily for the limited funds, both public and private, available to support good service programs. Increasingly, programs are finding that state and federal funding are less available for supporting existing service programs. Providers have had to create even tighter efficiencies and attempt to supplement public funds with private support. Since this is happening on such a broad scale, availability of this source of funding is diminishing as well.

The challenge, therefore, is to maximize accessibility to funding and to create a set of circumstances that increases the viability of the service in obtaining needed funding support. Several principles emerge in today's market that can be applied to this effort which can increase the chance that adequate funding support will be obtained:

- Find out the focus or emphasis of the funding source and incorporate that knowledge into the design of the funding proposal. This should be an honest effort to apply the relevant criteria for funding to the service for which it is being requested. If there is not a strong fit between funding source and funding proposal, it is likely that the funding source is not sound.

- Delineate the kinds of elements in the mission, purposes, or objectives of the funding source that relate directly to the work of the service entity. Maximize that relationship in the initial contact with the funder and clarify it in the proposal. Making that connection strengthens the chance of obtaining support.

- Never underestimate the effectiveness of relationships. More dollars are generated for a multitude of purposes based on the trust in and the quality of good relationships than any other single factor. The service provider must incorporate networking and relationship building with the funding community as an ongoing component of the leadership role. Access and availability to the funder increase the chance of being identified when money is being generated for service providers.

- Form coalitions with other involved or invested service providers. This consortium building is an excellent way to prove that you have networked with the service community to either share or maximize viability for receiving specified funding dollars. Often this integrated effort tells the funder that the service provider(s) are prepared to support each other, undertake a comprehensive approach to service provision, and effectively maximize dollars applied to the array of services represented by the coalition.

- There is nothing better than being in the right place at the right time. This is an operational process. The service provider cannot access what is not known. In each community there are times of the year when certain public and private funding processes are operating. The provider must become alert to the habits and patterns of the funders and be available at the right time to take advantage of the timing to make a request.

- Sometimes special funding opportunities may appear in the press or may be passed down by word of mouth. Being oriented to discerning these funding patterns assures that the provider has access to funding sources.

- The service provider must know that there are many funding sources that are not readily or easily identified. There are small granting agencies or departments in the federal and state governments that invariably have funds that should be accessed. More often, banks trusts and family or local community foundations have dollars which must be given away to the local community for purposes of providing service to the needy and underserved. Locating these and becoming cycled into the funding pattern of the foundation can often assure long-term viability and access to private funding.

- Staying connected with the funding source is a wise way of retaining the relationship. Exemplary are regular reports of how their money is being spent, reports on how coalition building is proceeding, anecdotes regarding the difference the donation is making, newsletters about the work, funder visits to the service agency, or anything that would keep a strong connection between the service provider and the funding body.

Learning the rules and patterns of funding behavior within the local community is essential to the role of the coalition leadership. The ability to remain solvent and viable as a service provider is important to those who count on service being provided. Building strong relationships and establishing an effective presence in the service and funding communities is one of the most important elements of successfully providing direct health service. Getting to know the local community and its resources and relationships, and strengthening them, can go a long way toward obtaining solid local support, a funding network, and broad-based commitment to nourish the activities of the service provider.

There are many benefits that accrue to building service coalitions. The ability to build comprehensive service structures, integrated quality improvement processes, better service measurement strategies and the ability to adjust services as the population changes and the demand for services shift. The leader of today must learn to develop integrated service models that involve others, create affiliation arrangements, and approach different ways of providing necessary services. Continuing economic constraints will drive all service processes to newer ways of building programs and providing assistance to those in need. Indeed, it is the challenge of the time.

REFERENCES

Beatty, J. (1990, February). A post cold war budget. *The Atlantic Monthly*, 74–82.

Lamm, R. (1991). A thousand flowers. *Health Management Quarterly, 13*(1), 7–10.

Porter-O'Grady, T., Patti, J., & McDonagh, K. (1990). *Streetside Support*, 60–62.

9

Nursing and Community Advocacy: Health Needs of the Young

Jeannette O. Poindexter

*I*n setting forth *The State of America's Children 1991,* the Children's Defense Fund observed, "America is at a crossroads of great national opportunity and danger. All of us, working together, must seize the opportunity to repair our nation's rent social fabric and ideals, and to save our endangered future" (Children's Defense Fund, p. 7). This is a tall order. When we look to the children and young people nearest to us, the next wave of essential adults needed to shoulder our nation's burdens, nurses must examine their role in the community as advocates on behalf of vulnerable populations who need committed professionals.

Existing abhorrent conditions associated with our infants, children, and adolescents represent a long term threat to the health and welfare of society. Statistical reports indicate:

- 12.6 million children now live below the poverty line.
- In 1984, 2 million children between the ages of 5 and 13 care for themselves after school.
- Infant mortality rate in the United States in one of the highest in industrialized nations.
- Five to 17-year-olds living in poverty lose 1.5 times more days of school than other students due to acute or chronic health conditions.
- Children living in poverty are twice as likely as affluent children to have health problems that impair daily activities.

- Black infant mortality in the United States ranks behind 31 other countries, including Hungary, Poland, and Cuba.
- In 1989, an estimated 7 million of the 28 million 10- to 17-year-old Americans were at risk of school failure, substance abuse, teen pregnancy and parenthood. Another 7 million were at moderate risk. Thus, half of American teens were at risk.
- Teens of families in poverty are three times as likely to drop out of school as other teens.
- One out of five adolescents has at least one serious health problem.
- One in seven adolescents has no health insurance.

The above list does not identify all of the many ills associated with the nation's next generation.

Advocacy, coalition-building, direct care, and policy formulation characterizes the nurse's involvement in the community on behalf of infants, children, and adolescents. Nurses involved in community efforts to improve the outcomes for this generation have found it necessary to increase their knowledge and skill in the areas of advocacy and coalition-building. They have learned to form networks with individuals and groups who have access to local, state, and national policy makers, as a basic foundation for bringing about changes. To implement and maintain effective programs in the community, knowledge and skills to access public and private sources of funding for programs and services for vulnerable populations are vital. Nurses who advocate on behalf of vulnerable populations, (1) identify an issue or target group, (2) become knowledgeable about the issues, (3) identify obstacles and positive forces, and (4) develop strategies to bring about changes.

Coalition-building can include individuals and organizations who work together using systematic approaches to improve the life and outcomes for at-risk-infants, children, and adolescents. As we know, nurses in the community work with individuals from different professional groups and lay organizations. Coalition membership usually reflects a variety of backgrounds and different areas of expertise. These individuals are committed to take the actions needed to bring about changes locally, regionally, and nationally.

Involved nurses must be knowledgeable about problems confronting adolescents and their families and have some understanding of the programs and services needed to assist them to make the transition to adulthood. The ability to network with groups who know how to build the needs and services of adolescents into the broad public agenda represents a basic requirement to support the vital connection between nurses and the community.

I have observed that advocacy activities in the community are initiated by making a commitment to a belief or a desire to make a difference in the community. As a maternal-child health nurse, I have been concerned about preventing adolescent pregnancies and promoting age-adequate adolescent growth and development. Both professional and community organizations provided a mechanism for my involvement with preadolescents, adolescents, and their families. I will summarize three projects to demonstrate how nurses can use their expertise to work with community groups to provide essential services for preadolescents, adolescents, and their families. The projects include: (1) implementation of a comprehensive school health course, (2) a training program for parents and their preadolescent and adolescents to delay early sexual involvement and pregnancy, and (3) provision of adolescent health services through school-based health centers.

In the first example, district school administrators and community leaders identified the need to implement a two-semester comprehensive school health course for 10th grade students during the early 1980s. The school administrators identified a committee of representatives from various interest groups in the school district. The committee included a nurse known for her involvement in the community with adolescent development workshops for parents and teachers.

The course content (see Table 1) and teaching aids were developed during regular monthly meetings. After about eight months, all materials were ready for approval.

All units, with the exception of "Unit IX: Human sexuality and reproductive health," were approved without difficulty by the school board and community groups. The unit on human sexuality and all of the teaching aids required further approval by the regional boards and the parent associations for each of the high schools in the district. The public health school nurse consultant and the nurse serving on the committee volunteered to present and discuss the human sexuality content and teaching aids with each of the five regional boards and the parent associations. It was extremely interesting to find that upon completion of the presentations, parents wanted workshops to learn more about human sexuality and reproductive health in order to discuss the content with their children. Parents also thought the content needed to be made available to their children in middle schools. It took almost a year to meet the requirements of approval for implementation of "Unit IX: Human sexuality and reproductive health."

The committee agreed to have the teachers and students evaluate the effectiveness of the course. An instrument was developed with the assistance of the school district researchers. The nurse's graduate students assisted with the analysis and writing of the report. When the school district found it necessary to decrease the required course from a two-semester course to a one-semester required course, the evaluation report was used to identify the content for the required course

Table 1
Personal Health Management Course

Unit and Title		Content
Unit I	Personal health assessment	Health needs inventory, health history, exercise survey, diet
Unit II	Personal health practices	Dental diseases, ears, eyes, skin problems, sleep and rest
Unit III	Disease prevention and control	Infectious disease process, acute and chronic diseases, communicable diseases, venereal disease, high blood pressure
Unit IV	Utilization of community health resources	EMS services, health career opportunities, community health organizations
Unit V	Utilization of health products	Health care products, attitude survey on substance abuse, advertising campaigns
Unit VI	First aid and personal safety	Poisoning, respiratory failure, drug overdose, fractures, CPR
Unit VII	Emotional/social health	Personality traits, nonverbal communications, body talk, emotional stress
Unit VIII	Parenting	Marriage contract, counseling, needs of the baby
Unit IX	Health sexuality and reproductive health	Sex roles, sexism, adolescent development, contraception

and the elective course. Almost eight years later, these two options remain in most of the district high schools.

A second example of community involvement can be found in the experiences of the nurse serving on the board of a community service organization for single parents and families. As a member of the board, with grant writing experiences, she shared information related to a call for proposals on pregnancy prevention in adolescents with the executive director. The nurse worked with the director of the agency to submit a proposal. The project, Delaying Early Sexual Involvement and Pregnancy (DESIP), was approved and funded. DESIP assists parents to become sex educators for their children by increasing their knowledge of growth and development and communication skills. Their preadolescent and adolescent children participate in seminars to assist them to deal with their sexuality and improve communication skills with their parents. To avoid conflict of interest, the nurse resigned from the board of directors to serve as project evaluator.

The final example is the development of a school-based health center in the local high schools. The nurse in this project is a member of the Detroit Black Nurses Association. The Detroit Black Nurses Association is a member of a coalition of black organizations, the Detroit Association of Black Organizations (DABO). DABO called upon its constituent organizations to support the development and implementation of a school-based health service center in the Detroit high schools. DABO's members, along with the other organizational members, provided information to the community to help inform parents and community leaders of the need for health services in the high schools. DABO formed a coalition with additional organizations to secure public and private funding to support the implementation of school-based health service centers in selected high schools.

The school-based health centers serve several thousand adolescents each year. An equal number of male and female adolescents receive services in the following categories:

- Chronic disease management
- Family planning
- Health promotion and risk reduction
- General medical
- Immunizations
- Mental health service and counseling
- Prenatal and postpartum care
- STD diagnosis and treatment
- Substance abuse diagnosis and treatment

A review of the annual school-based health center's reports indicates that 70 to 80 percent of adolescents are receiving general medical services. Mental health services and family planning are similar in number and account for about 10 percent of the services delivered. Clinical nurse specialists are the primary providers of services in these centers. There is no question that the adolescents are using these centers to meet their health care needs.

Adolescents and their families are dependent on nurses to set up approaches to care that will provide the most cost effective and best direct care services. Nursing educational programs are expected to prepare providers who are familiar with children and adolescent health problems and needs. Therefore, the challenge is to increase the number of nurses prepared for the needs of children and adolescents.

Individuals cannot contribute to society if they do not receive support to develop healthy minds and bodies. As our young people struggle with the results of poor health care, they recognize that the people entrusted with the distribution of public resources are not considering their needs as priorities. Yes, they are bitter, and sometimes unable to help themselves and others, but they are not hopeless. With our advocacy, young people will not continue to live with conditions which leave them unable to contribute to the health and welfare for themselves and society when they become adults.

REFERENCES

Children's Defense Fund. *The state of America's children 1991.* (1991). Washington, DC: Author.

Mesce, D. (1991, April 2). An unhealthy group of U.S. kids. *Detroit News.*

10

A Church-Based Program for the Homeless

Cora Newell-Withrow

The plight of homeless citizens is a national disgrace. Homeless citizens suffer many complex health problems (e.g., chronic skin lesions and infections, hypertension, ulcers, respiratory diseases, heart problems, and diabetes). Homeless children may have experienced abuse and neglect. They may be easily susceptible to communicable diseases because of missed and incomplete immunizations (Lindsey, 1989). It is believed that mental illness affects one third of this population (Hodnicki, 1990). Malloy, Christ, and Hohlock (1990) reported that 84 percent of the homeless have psychiatric diagnoses. Drug and alcohol abuse are also a major problem which can result in more health problems, as well as conflicts with the law.

When the homeless attempt to seek health care, they experience barriers; they have little or no money to pay for care and often are confronted with uncaring attitudes from health professionals (McDonald, 1986). The homeless may avoid seeking health care or fail in trying, because of the complexity of the system. Most services are not located within areas of their daily travel, which in turn creates more confusion for them (McDonald, 1986). Perhaps more importantly, health care is not always a top priority for them, especially when their efforts may be focused on where to obtain their next meal and where to sleep.

CLINICAL PRACTICE

To determine what is needed in clinical practice arenas, I would like to share my story. Our church-based program began in 1985. Its purpose was to strengthen existing community services. We knew that our efforts resembled the bandaid approach to the complex social and health problems suffered by the homeless. Nevertheless, we consciously decided to take this approach rather than doing nothing.

The plight of people without food and shelter was brought to my attention by a local police inspector. He was concerned about the people without food and shelter, especially the aged and children. He proposed at the time that churches needed to be more responsive to the needs of people. He also wanted to know what could be done about the problem. How could we motivate churches to take the initiative? We decided at the time to start by approaching one church.

A proposal was presented, accepted, and supported by the church membership. The uniqueness of this church was that its membership consisted of approximately 60 percent retirees. Of these, 40 percent were living entirely on social security benefits, with incomes of less than $400.00 per month. Members, however, supported this program and made financial contributions. (For example, one 78-year-old member saves nickels and dimes all summer in order to support the program.)

The program was to be offered from October through April of each year. Services were to be delivered from the church's van parked on a specified lot where large numbers of homeless citizens congregate each night. Services were to include food, clothing, small travel kits (with a toothbrush, toothpaste, soap, and a wash cloth), referrals, education, and someone with whom to talk.

Most of the target population was transient and included men, women, and children of all races. About 5 percent of this population had families living in the community. Those homeless with family members in the community who could help them were often estranged, primarily due to chronic drug abuse and mental illness. The majority of the women were of childbearing age. Less than 2 percent were pregnant; those who were pregnant received sporadic prenatal care or no care at all. The children, according to their mothers, suffered primarily from URIs, had incomplete immunization records, poor school attendance, and problems with learning. The senior population consisted primarily of males age 55 and older. They complained of, for example, heart problems, hypertension, problems with feet and legs, and alcohol abuse. It was very clear when it was the first of the month, because of the increased incidences of alcohol abuse. People tended to take only the clothing they needed. They were quick to return clothing if they thought someone else was worse off. They tended to look out for the children when it was time to eat and they always talked about going home.

Another characteristic of importance was social isolation. It was expressed by some of the homeless citizens in the following statements: "I would love to walk up the road and have people really look at me." "I guess it's because I smell and look funny that people look scared."

My question was, "Do you think if you would remove some of your outer layers of clothes that you would not appear so different?" The response was "No, because I ain't got no place to put my clothes except on me." Alternatively "I am going home tomorrow as soon as I get my social security check." Often, after making this statement, this same gentlemen would assume a position in the middle of the lawn and quietly talk to his deceased mother.

The number of people we served depended on the weather. For example, if the temperature dropped to 30° or below, our count on a given evening was 100 people. If the temperature was above 30°, our count was usually no more than 50 people. One cannot do this type of work without a sense of humor. For example, for two weeks we had an increase in the number of adolescent males and we were not sure why this was occurring. We later discovered that these young people were coming from basketball practice and they thought they would stop and have a snack. Another example was our minister who loved to preach about caring for the poor and disabled. One night the minister was asked for his coat to give to one of our homeless guests, when he said without thinking, "It's cold. What will I do?", our response was, "You have a car, keys, and a heater in your car. We will now receive your jacket. Amen!"

WHAT DOES THE FUTURE HOLD?

There are four major areas of concern in a community program for the homeless: education, research, practice, and access.

Education

We must shape the nursing curricula using public health and community health models. These models would address the health objectives planned for the nation for the year 2000. We must also change the focus of leadership and management courses in nursing education. The change would include concepts and practice of the management of care. It is important that students have the opportunity to have reality-based learning experiences that integrate theory and practice (Witt, 1981). It is also important to place greater emphasis on collaboration, risk-taking, assertiveness, decision-making, and critical thinking.

Research for the Future

Research about the homeless is essential. Tracking systems, as an outgrowth of research, that monitor people need to be developed. (Stephen et al., 1990). We must produce empirical data that provide information about subgroups within the homeless population (1990). We must discover cost effective health promotion programs and ways to teach about self-care and self-advocacy. Databases that contribute to systematic planning and execution of health services need to be established.

Future Practice Needs

If the use of case managers and management of care methodologies are strategies for the future, we must not be overzealous in service agencies by depriving students of opportunities that would allow them to learn. Educators and service personnel must strengthen collaborative efforts. We must somehow arrive at an understanding of how we can help each other in the education of professional nurses.

In the practice arenas, nurses working with the homeless must tune their skill as practitioners and advocates. In addition, they must develop in their role as health educators by teaching the homeless how to become more independent and assertive.

Access

Access to health care is a current and future concern. Because of the complexity of health and social problems of homeless citizens, a single approach, such as the one described in this chapter will not suffice. Collaborative efforts with emphasis on proactive strategies are required from the social, economic, political and health sectors to jointly address health and social problems that affect the lives of our citizens to the extent that they are forced to live on the streets. Nurses are the appropriate professionals to lead this positive action.

RATIONING OF HEALTH CARE

In the future, rationing health care will become more of a concern and reality. Therefore, we must now begin to discuss the following questions:

1. What does it mean morally and ethically to ration health care?
2. Will we have to make decisions that will determine who will or will not receive treatment? If so, who will decide?
3. Will we opt against costly high-tech treatments for specified populations in place of less costly treatment for all?

4. Will we provide health care for the homeless on a limited bases because they are considered nonproductive members of our society?

5. Will we make a concerted effort to plan programs that address health promotion, wellness, and prevention of disease?

REFERENCES

Hodnicki, D. R. (1990). "Homeless: Healthcare implications." *Journal of Community Health Nursing, 7* (2), 59–67.

Malloy, C., Christ, M. A., & Hohlock, F. J. (1990). "The homeless: Social isolates." *Journal of Community Health Nursing, 7* (1), 25–36.

Witt, B. S. (1991). "The homeless shelter: An ideal clinical setting for RN/BSN students." *Nursing and Health Care, 12* (6), 304–307.

11

Prevention as the Intervention of Choice

Mae E. Markstrom and Kathryn Fiandt

Our community-based project, the Wellness CARE Center, funded by the W. K. Kellogg Foundation in 1988 and 1990, is a nurse-directed model of health care delivery which serves the citizens in the Eastern Upper Peninsula of Michigan. This three-county, rural, underserved area is larger than the states of Delaware, Rhode Island, and the District of Columbia combined, encompassing 3520 square miles. The Wellness CARE Center is part of the department of health sciences at Lake Superior State University, a small, public university in Sault Ste. Marie, Michigan, on the Canadian border. The primary location of the Wellness CARE Center is in the Medical Building next to the local hospital in downtown Sault Ste. Marie.

The CARE acronym represents four major types of services offered by the nursing center: (1) consultation, (2) advocacy, (3) referral, and (4) education services. The purposes of the Wellness CARE Centers are: (1) to provide holistic, wellness oriented nursing care to clients of all ages in the area, (2) to provide a clinical site for faculty and student practice, and (3) to provide an environment for practitioners, faculty, and students to engage in research.

The Center's health care team is composed of nursing staff, nursing faculty, university students, and consultants. The clinical director is the nurse executive. She has primary accountability for overall functioning of the nursing center. She provides advanced practice services as a family nurse practitioner. She also supervises clinical practice, program activities, and the development and implementation of research proposals. Professional nurses provide nursing services, health education, screening services, and participate in research and program implementation. An exercise science specialist provides clients with exercise fitness prescriptions as well as health education and adds an interdisciplinary dimension to the staff. An administrative assistant, who is responsible for office management, budget management, and marketing, a receptionist, and university work study students compose the office staff. In addition, nursing faculty from the university have special assignments at the Center. Faculty practice is voluntary and is not required by the university. These clinical nurse specialists provide services in their respective disciplinary areas. A nutritionist is employed on a contractual basis, and a family practitioner physician is hired part-time as a medical consultant to review advanced practice services.

The Wellness CARE Center is structured within the organizational framework of Lake Superior State University. The project director is the head of the university's department of health sciences. This structure has been beneficial to the Center as administration and faculty are very supportive of the project. The Center receives organizational support from university experts who assist with computer operations, legal counsel, research and evaluation, accounting, and personnel management.

The community is a major part of the Center's operation. Staff involvement in community activities facilitates access to information regarding unmet community health needs and opportunities to disseminate information regarding Center's activities within the community. The Center uses an interdisciplinary approach to many of its programs which promotes group collaboration. Overall, ongoing collaboration between provider agencies has been an important component of our project. This has promoted good interpersonal and interagency relationships which has helped the Center to become a valuable participant of health care delivery in the Eastern Upper Peninsula.

The Center maintains a community advisory committee consisting of both consumers and professional health care providers. The functions of the committee are to provide input and suggestions for operation of the Center, to identify health care needs of the target population, and to participate in public relations and fund raising projects for the Center.

In 1988, the Kellogg Foundation awarded Lake Superior State University a three year grant to establish an ambulatory nursing center and rural health services for the population age 60 or older in the Eastern Upper Peninsula. According to the 1990 census, there are approximately 10,000 seniors age 60 or older living in the area. Of this population, 40 percent are estimated to have unmet health needs. Our rural elderly population experience multiple problems impacting upon their health status; these include social isolation, transportation difficulties, limited access to health services and health care providers, poverty, deteriorating housing, and increased accidents.

The purpose of our project was to protect, sustain, and restore the ability of the elderly population to maintain independence by reducing the risk of injury, disease, and deterioration of health. Thus, the primary focus of our health services is health promotion and maintenance, and the prevention of illness. Health services are offered to senior citizens in collaboration with the Chippewa-Luce-Mackinac Community Action Agency, a state-funded agency providing a variety of helping services to the elderly. This affiliation has provided the Center access to 19 senior nutrition sites. Our staff brings professional nursing services to sites located throughout the area, including three island sites accessible only by ferry or plane. The major problem with this affiliation is that all senior citizens do not participate in Community Action activities, including seniors living in residential complexes and foster care homes, those not near nutrition sites, and others who may have a personal bias against low-income and social service programs.

In February of 1991, the Kellogg Foundation awarded Lake Superior State University three additional years of funding. The grant has two major objectives, the first being to expand the Center's services for adults age 60 or older. The staff has worked with both well and frail elderly adults in the community for the past three years. During this time, senior clients have responded well to education regarding their health status and have actively participated in program activities. Research studies have been conducted concerning client utilization of the nursing center; cholesterol screening, monitoring, and education; and the effectiveness of exercise on client mobility. Positive outcomes in decreasing cholesterol levels and increasing joint mobility and range of motion have been demonstrated. While this project has been successful, expanding our senior program will allow the staff to provide additional health care services to elderly adults—with an emphasis on increasing knowledge and skills needed for developing self-care behaviors, training community grassroots leaders, and improving access to health care.

The second objective of the Kellogg grant is to extend services to midlife adults 40 years of age and older. Adults at midlife face multiple developmental tasks, often including responsibility for the care of an aging parent. This responsibility is sometimes combined with the continued responsibility of child-rearing and employment. As a result of these multiple demands of children, parents, and employment, today's midlife adults are described as the sandwich generation who often neglect their own self-care. Healthy diets, regular exercise, and routine health screening are considered low priority. The purpose of this grant is to develop accessible programs to assist midlife adults in developing and maintaining healthy life-styles and in promoting a healthy, successful aging process.

We believe that rural nursing centers affiliated with academic institutions provide quality health care services to underserved rural populations who usually have a high incidence of chronic illness and poverty. The services provided by our nursing center are valuable to our community and provide a method of health care delivery congruent with Nursing's Agenda for Health Care Reform. The Wellness CARE Center provides primary health care services geared toward promoting, restoring, and maintaining health and wellness. The staff encourage client responsibility for health care decision through collaboration between consumers and providers. Our interventions are client oriented; we go to the client and try to work within the client's reality. Clients play an active role in health care and are encouraged to take responsibility for developing and maintaining healthy lifestyles. Our interdisciplinary approach to health care provides increased consumer access to quality health care services which are appropriate, effective, cost-efficient, and focused on consumer needs.

The Wellness CARE Center meets the guidelines set forth for nursing centers in *The Nursing Center: Concept and Design.* Our Center provides the client with direct access to nursing services. Using a nursing model based upon Neuman and Orem's, our professional nurses assess, diagnose, and treat actual and potential health problems. Health care services are consumer oriented and reimbursable. Our professional nurses accept full accountability for their nursing practice with overall responsibility assumed by the clinical director of the Center.

After years of work at the Center, we have learned important lessons affecting the success of a nursing center.

1. Staff needs to be optimistic, future oriented, flexible, and willing to make changes.

2. Health care needs must be identified by the clients, not the provider, with grassroots community leaders playing a key role in this process.

3. Consumer education must not only focus upon health maintenance and promotion, but also on the development of motivation for client self-care.

4. Health care services must be provided on an ongoing cycle, with specific schedules identified and marketed widely in local communities.

5. There is a major need to develop good marketing strategies to communicate nursing services as valued health care services to both consumers and other health care providers.

6. Ongoing collaboration with other health care agencies and providers must be an major component of nursing center projects.

University students play a very important role in the functioning of a nursing center. Practitioners provide excellent role models for these future health care providers. During the past year, university students have received over 1300 hours of clinical experience at the Center. The success of the Center has been largely due to the community, which is very open to change and to new strategies for delivery of health care. It has also been important to have the university's support to facilitate implementation of the project. Finally, we need to communicate our successes to both our professional community and the public and assist our colleagues in developing nursing models of health care delivery. Long-term goals of the Center are: (1) to become a self-sufficient nursing center, (2) to offer primary health care services which reduce the incidence and costs of chronic illness, (3) to facilitate successful, healthy aging, and (4) to encourage consumer self-care and independence.

We live in a rapidly changing society with new opportunities emerging for professional nurses in health care delivery. Smith (1987) states:

> Where there is change and uncertainty, there is also opportunity. Today a whole new set of career opportunities is available in nursing. The future belongs to the visionary—to those who can create new configurations to respond to new demands and who have the courage to follow their vision. (p. 42)

EVALUATION

In June of 1990, as a part of the review process for the writing of our second Kellogg grant, the Center staff updated our annual goals to reflect our expansion from a seniors' focus to an age 40 or older focus. For 1990-91 our goals included expanding our seniors' program, health education program, worksite wellness program, and advocacy services. We also planned to initiate a midlife program. In conjunction with our program goals we developed some process goals, specifically, to improve our program development process, implement our program evaluation process, improve our marketing, and continue to support university education and research goals. We also developed outcome goals: to demonstrate increased self-sufficiency and increased utilization. We have been highly successful in achieving our 1990-91 goals.

Although we offer some medical model services (e.g., treatment of minor illnesses) we are committed to implementing a model based on a nursing philosophy. We use an eclectic approach to theory-based practice and see our interventions as grounded in multiple theoretical models. Our advanced practice is, of course, based somewhat in the medical model. Many of our interventions, however, such as foot care and ear irritations in our elderly clients, are based on Orem's self-care nursing model. Our mental health services are grounded in a variety of psychosocial models and our health education is based, in large part, on a semiotic model of health education developed by the Center's clinical director. We are also using Pender's health promotion model as the organizing framework for a community-based health needs assessment. The underlying belief of this approach is that independent nursing practice models must be derived from paradigmatic alternatives to the medical model in order to support the idea that we are offering truly alternative health care services.

The Center has multiple ongoing activities. Many of these programs are offered to clients of all ages, although the focus of the services is the midlife and senior adult. Our first group of programs are health education. Many of the programs are offered in collaboration with the local hospital (e.g., diabetic education) and through the university's continuing education program (e.g., wellness for women and assertiveness). Participation in these programs numbers in the hundreds of clients per year.

The Center offers many traditional advanced practice services. These services are provided by nurse practitioners, psychiatric clinical nurse specialists, and our American College of Sports Medicine certified health and fitness instructor. As mentioned earlier, we have a physician consultant who reviews our illness practice monthly and has delegated prescription privileges to our nurse practitioners. Our illness practice is a primary source of income, especially as we begin to receive reimbursement through Medicaid, Medicare, and CHAMPUS. We believe, however, that our illness practice is secondary and functions to allow us access to clients to whom we can offer nursing wellness services.

We offer screenings of cholesterol, glucose, blood pressure, and hearing. This is primarily a community support service and we travel with these services to many locations in the area. We also travel with our nursing services; we have conducted nursing clinics in schools, churches, community centers, and fire stations. These services are also taken to homebound clients, particularly foot care and flu shots.

Our worksite wellness program is our primary access to the midlife adult, a real expression of Nursing's Agenda for Health Care Reform. Thus far this year, we have conducted health risk appraisals for over 800 people at seven different worksites. We have taken exercise classes, weight control programs, and health education classes into these worksites. Employers are supportive and will usually give one-half hour off per session in exchange for one-half hour of the employee's time.

As the Center is located in a sparsely populated, rural area, we travel to 19 different nutrition centers to provide screening services to seniors. We also take our services to fixed locations where there are limited or no primary care services. We conduct women's clinics and have offered semi-permanent primary care services in the small community of Pickford and on Drummond Island. We hope to expand these services to other small towns in the future.

Payment for services is a critical concern given our goal of self-sufficiency. Many of our services are fee-for-service. We find that even insured clients do not have insurance that will cover many of our services (e.g., foot care in the healthy senior). As a result we charge limited fees (e.g., $10 for a one-half hour to one hour foot care appointment). Third party reimbursement is coming; we have had CHAMPUS and Medicaid since June 1, 1991. We also anticipate Medicare as we qualify as a rural setting. The university is working with its health insurance provider, Blue Cross and Blue Shield of Michigan, and is requesting direct reimbursement for nurse practitioners who offer covered services. The Michigan Nurses' Association has been very supportive throughout the state in efforts to receive third party reimbursement for services.

As a part of our new Kellogg grant we are conducting a major community-based health needs assessment. The purposes of the needs assessment are: to describe the health status of our population, to identify the health related behaviors of our population, and to identify the image of the Wellness CARE Center in the three-county area. We are receiving support for this project from the University's Center for Social Research. We started the process by looking for an organizational framework for our data collection. We chose Pender's health promotion model (1982) for two major reasons. First, the model identifies factors we see as influencing our clients' health care behavior. Second, it is a nursing model. The model, derived from the health belief model, identifies a series of cognitive-perceptual and modifying factors which are assumed to influence health promotion behavior. We assumed that our theory-based interventions served as cues to action in the model. We had identified as our population adults in the three-county area. We needed, therefore, to sample an appropriate representation of a population of approximately 30,000 people.

Following identification of an organizational framework and articulation of our population, we identified a series of research questions that would address Pender's health promotion factors. We also identified data that would be most appropriate to address each question. The questions were:

1. *"What are the health behaviors of the population?"* Health behaviors are a factor in Pender's model. We will use our health risk appraisal data for this question and are preparing a questionnaire to distribute throughout the community.

2. *"What is the health status of the population?"* This question reflects Pender's perceived health status, biological characteristics, and demographics factors. We are using health risk appraisal data, 1990 area census data, and Michigan public health data to address this question.

3. *"What are the perceived and actual barriers to health care?"* Barriers to health care are included in situational factors, interpersonal influences, and perceived benefits and barriers to health-promoting behavior in Pender's model. We are using some Michigan public health data to identify access problems. We are collecting information regarding social support and responsibilities concurrent with our health risk appraisal data and in our communitywide questionnaire. In addition, we will be conducting interviews with area residents to collect data addressing this question.

4. *"What are the population's beliefs about health and health care?"* This question addresses the importance of health, perceived control of health, perceived self-efficacy, and definition of health as factors in Pender's model. Some clients at the Center are completing Laffrey's health conception scale (1986) as an assessment of the definition of health based on Smith's (1983) categories (e.g., clinical, functional, adaptive, and eudiamonistic). Additional data will be collected in interviews.

In addition to health needs assessment data, we are collecting data from a marketing perspective. The two marketing questions are: (1) *"What is the level of satisfaction of our clients?"* and (2) *"What is the image of the Center in the community?"* We have mailed a client satisfaction questionnaire to all clients of the Center with health records. Of 389 questionnaires mailed, 126 were returned complete. Questions regarding the image of the Center are a part of the questionnaire mailed to the community.

We will use collected information to construct a thumbnail sketch of our population to support current programs, in planning future programming, and in marketing our services to the community. We also hope to use the information for program evaluation and plan to replicate the data collection process following expansion of services in the future.

Ongoing program evaluation, like research, is often difficult to conduct in the rush of our everyday activities. We have, however, developed standards for evaluation work toward accessing how well we meet each one annually. (The standards are listed in Table 1.) Evidence of these standards has been threaded throughout this presentation. We believe that in order for nursing centers such as ours to become a viable part of the health care system we must meet the standards listed, must document the efficacy of our practice, and must market our services throughout our communities. The staff of the Wellness CARE Center have made a commitment to achieving these goals. We have found the barriers rather daunting, but have learned that the barriers are often a result of our own limited thinking or unwillingness to commit to risk-taking behavior. Every time we overcome these internal barriers we have met success.

Table 1
Wellness CARE Center Standards of Practice

Standard I   Philosophy, purpose, goals
There are clearly stated philosophy, purpose, and goals for the provision of service.

Standard II   Organizational structure
There is a current written plan describing the organization structure.

Standard III   Administration
Nursing services are under the direction of a legally and educationally qualified nurse who is responsible to the Kellogg Project director.

Standard IV   Functional support
There is adequate space, facilities, and equipment to support the clinical and educational functions of the center.

Standard V   Policies, procedures, protocols
There are current, written policies, procedures, and advanced practice protocols to describe the scope and function of nursing practice.

Standard VI   Quality assurance
There is evidence that client's needs are being assessed and that services provided are consistent with those needs and are within standards of written procedures and protocols.

Standard VII   Professional development
Wellness CARE center staff participate in formal and informal continuing education activities to improve knowledge and skill.

Standard VIII   Program development
Program planning is based on the center's philosophy and purpose and is supported by health needs assessment research.

Standard IX   Program evaluation
There is an evaluation program in place which includes ongoing needs assessment, documentation of practice efficacy, and research.

We are convinced that the nursing center model is the best possible future for health care in this country. We also believe that nurses, especially university-based nurses with the skill and knowledge resources needed, should commit to initiating and supporting the nursing center model in their community.

REFERENCES

Laffrey, S. C. (1986). Development of a health conception scale. *Research in Nursing and Health, 9,* 107–113.

Pender, N. J. (1982). *Health promotion in nursing.* East Norwalk, CT: Appleton-Century-Crofts.

Smith, G. R. (1987). The new health care economy: Opportunities for nurse entrepreneurs. *Nursing Outlook, 35* (4), 40–42.

Smith, J. A. (1983). *The idea of health.* New York: Teachers College Press.

PART FIVE

Distance Education and New Technology

12

Distance Education: Turf and Technology

Myrna R. Pickard

The University of Texas at Arlington School of Nursing has had a strong mission in rural health since its inception in 1971. Rural outreach and continuing education were first offered in 1975 and continue to this time. In 1985, in cooperation with East Texas State University in Texarkana and the Texarkana Community College, an outreach campus for the RN to BSN program was initiated in Texarkana. The community requested the opening of an outreach campus due to the difficulty in hiring qualified faculty to teach in all subject areas. Community leaders from Texarkana met with faculty from The University of Texas at Arlington (UTA) in 1988 to consider offering nursing courses via telecommunication and satellite and using flexible, innovative, and creative approaches to increase the number of professional nurses in that geographical location. Through the combined efforts of the community and UTA, a Special Projects Grant (D10 NU 26156-01) from the Department of Health and Human Services for a Nursing Education Telecommunication Satellite System was submitted and funded.

INITIATION OF PROJECT

Turf and Technology in Distance Learning began in earnest in June, 1990. Planning the technical action for activating the system had to be completed in three months as the first broadcast was scheduled for September, 1990. We were fortunate in having a faculty member prepared to serve as technical director. We also hired a small business firm to do a turnkey job by contract. The vendor would supply all engineering hardware, software, delivery, installation, site coordination, licensing, proof of performance testing, and, any other necessities to deliver a working system by our deadline. We included maintenance, evaluation, and ongoing consultation in the contract. Our objective was to establish the satellite telecommunication network to deliver the nursing curriculum to designated rural areas: Texarkana, Waco, Paris, and Sherman. For the initial phase, we have restricted distance education to the accelerated RN to BSN curriculum plan. Our goal is to increase the number of BSN prepared nurses to meet the health needs in rural areas.

TECHNICAL REQUIREMENTS AND RESOURCES

We had planned to purchase a microwave dish, but the cost exceeded the grant request. Instead, we substituted a three-year rental agreement with the option to buy at the end of the grant period. Our broadcasts are delivered, by a microwave link, from The University of Texas at Arlington campus to the Dallas–Fort Worth Teleport—to a geostationary satellite. The satellite links the signal to the receiving sites. In fact, anyone in North America with a satellite dish can receive our broadcasts as they are not scrambled. Receiving sites need downlink receptors and a dedicated telephone line. UTA School of Nursing already had a fully equipped television studio. A semicircular teaching station was purchased with connections for audio hookup with a control room, allowing one to control slides and the overhead camera shots of printed material. Besides, there was adequate space for sitting, standing, walking around, and guests.

As we considered technical requirements and resources, we decided to have a remote-controlled camera rather than one operated by faculty. The short timeframe for faculty preparation was part of the rationale underlying that decision. We also wanted faculty to feel comfortable with the teaching station. We felt it was important to have a live, warm human being in the studio. This proved to be a valuable stress reduction measure. Other requirements included time-based correctors, computer interface, lighting, backup microphones, a telephone setup, carpeting, and set design. An overhead graphics camera, clocks, a character generator, and a way to communicate with the technical director were also necessary. Interactive communication was accomplished through telephone contact from the sites and transmitted via the control room to the on air instructor. Instant feedback was an important feature of our distance learning.

FACULTY NEEDS

I am frequently asked how faculty adjust to and accept telecommunications. As with any new teaching strategy, there is some initial anxiety.

Faculty need ventilation time, preparation time, a workshop, reality time, and flexibility. They definitely need graphic support and instructional design ideas. They need to become aware of color of clothing, makeup techniques, and body language. These needs were addressed through a week long workshop to assist faculty, giving them an opportunity to practice with the equipment.

At the beginning of the workshop, faculty identified their concerns about TV teaching. These concerns were reviewed at the conclusion of the workshop and found to be less significant. Major themes of the instructional workshop included: to be prepared, to be organized, to give the technician a plan prior to the broadcast, and to do a dry run with the technician prior to the broadcast.

The most common comment from faculty was regarding the time needed for preparation. Teaching via satellite requires more structure in the presentations than in classroom teaching. Timing has to be perfect. Faculty also indicated that personal contact with remote sites and students was essential. Each instructor needs to make at least one site visit while their course is taught.

The last phase of the workshop was preparing faculty for imperfection. They are not supposed to become television stars. Spontaneity and promoting lively discussions are more important. Each teaching session was followed with debriefing, review, and sharing.

STUDENT RESPONSE

All of our students are either associate degree or diploma students pursuing a baccalaureate degree in an accelerated program. They are able to complete the upper division nursing courses in two semesters rather than four. While the majority of their classes are via telecommunication, some are taught on site. Students were asked to evaluate their first year; there was overall satisfaction with the program. Many indicated they would not have been able to enroll in school without telecommunication. For them, it was beneficial to save on transportation costs to the UTA campus. Also many had family responsibilities and could not spare the time for commuting. Students stated that the lack of immediacy was counter-balanced through the interaction with the site coordinator at the end of each class. Students believed that because of greater organization the quality of instruction via telecommunication was better than in regular classroom. They requested more handouts. They wanted the instructor to continue to come to their campus at the beginning of each course.

Students also requested that we should present the programs live with on-campus students at The University of Texas at Arlington. We had not done this the first year because of the need to dedicate efforts toward off campus sites. Live classroom broadcasts will be presented next year.

Students had one other suggestion regarding the time framework. They found that four straight hours of telecommunications was too long. Consequently, they requested that we broadcast two hours in the morning, with an hour break, and two hours in the afternoon. Students' comments on graphics, such as overheads and video presentations, were positive.

COSTS AND CONTINUATION

It is always an issue to decide on the continuation of telecommunications because of high equipment and satellite transmission costs. The total grant for implementing this project over a three-year period was $780,000. The transmission costs are about $610 per hour and the schools' projected total cost for the hours transmitted the next academic year will be $66,000. There is also the expense of paying site coordinators at each location to clarify technical questions and to assist with the teaching activities.

Data are being collected to look at similarities and differences in campus and satellite learners. Data regarding cost per semester hour to the institution are also being collected and analyzed. Continuation will depend upon locating adequate financing. Organizations are offered the opportunity to purchase time to communicate recruitment or sponsorship messages to nurses across Texas and the nation. There are four ten-minute break periods available for purchase during each broadcast. We have also considered leasing the studio to other departments. We shall continue looking at alternative funding and alternative systems.

SUMMARY

Distance learning fits with the mission and strategic plan of The University of Texas at Arlington. We believe these educational opportunities in nursing are highly desirable. The Board of Nurse Examiners for the State of Texas has approved this project and the Texas Higher Education Coordinating Board has approved it as a pilot project. The school will continue evaluation and creative problem-solving in the use of distance education.

ACKNOWLEDGMENTS

The author wishes to acknowledge four colleagues who have made this project possible: Dr. Wanda Thompson, Associate Professor and Project Director, UTA; Dr. Mary Ellen Wyers, Professor and Associate Dean, UTA; Norman "Pat" Patrick, Technical Director and Specialist, UTA; and Dr. Myrna Armstrong, Associate Professor, UTA.

13

Distant Learning in Nursing

Michael A. Carter

The purpose of this chapter is to discuss some of the more technical aspects of distant learning, particularly as these might apply to teaching nursing at the undergraduate and graduate levels. Distant learning is not a new concept, but is relatively new in nursing. Because at last we have concluded that we cannot place a nursing school in every location that needs one, an interest in distant learning has begun to develop in nursing schools. In Tennessee, this lesson may be too late. Tennessee has almost 43 different RN programs and 38 LPN programs, most receiving state assistance in some form, most not fully subscribed, and most having difficulty attracting and retaining faculty in the desired numbers and quality. This chapter provides an overview of some of the different types of distant learning approaches available to schools of nursing today, followed by a description of the approach being used at Tennessee's health science center.

FORMS OF DISTANT LEARNING

Distant learning is an educational approach in which the learner is not in the same location as the teacher. There are a number of forms this type of education can take, but, generally, these can be described as: (1) one-way learning, (2) partial two-way learning, and (3) full two-way learning.

One-Way Learning

One-way learning is characterized by the teacher providing information to the student, without the student being able to communicate back to the teacher, at least, in real time. Exemplary of one-way learning is the use of self-study programs of written, audio, or audio-video materials. In this format there is little student-to-student or student-to-teacher interaction. When interaction does take place, it is in the form of mail, fax, or phone calls. This form of learning is useful for the communication of information that is primarily factual such as that seen in a number of college level, didactic courses. Courses such as nursing theory, legal aspects of nursing, statistics, pathophysiology, and research methods lend themselves to one-way learning.

Partial Two-Way Learning

Partial two-way learning is a form of distant learning in which the student and teacher interact in real time, but without full audio and video capabilities. Examples of this include two-way audio by means of conference telephone calls or one-way video, and two-way audio learning situations.

Conference calls to multiple sites require the use of an electronic bridging device. This device modulates all incoming and outgoing calls to make sure they are at similar audio levels. These devices connect to the switch of the phone system, either the college's or the phone company's, and are simple to use. Calls can be initiated from within the college utilizing the WATS line or by students utilizing their personal billing number.

One-way video and two-way audio adds images of the teacher to the learning situation. There are generally two approaches to this type of distant learning. One is the use of microwave transmissions. The other one is the use of satellite uplink and receiving stations. Both of these approaches require telephone connections back to the teacher for two-way audio transmission.

Full Two-Way Learning

Full two-way learning requires much more sophisticated transmission and receiving equipment at both the teaching and learning locations. There are three approaches. One is an expansion of the microwave system that allows reception and transmission from each site. A second approach is the use of satellite uplinks and downlinks at two or more sites. A third approach, one that is growing rapidly, is the use of compressed video, interactive conferencing. Compressed video utilizes existing telephone lines to send and receive images, voice, and data at the same time.

ADVANTAGES AND DISADVANTAGES

The primary advantage of one-way learning formats is that they are relatively inexpensive to produce and distribute and are widely available. Audio and audiovideo tapes can be sent anywhere there is mail service. The equipment needed for their playback is available in almost every home. The programs may be utilized at times convenient to the learner and replayed as often as desired.

The major disadvantages of one-way learning formats is that there is no real time communication between the teacher and the learner. Any visual materials selected by the teacher must be prepared well ahead and sent to the learner prior to the learning experience. This format makes it difficult for the teacher to determine the immediate learner's response to the materials and to clarify or amplify any points the learner does not understand.

The advantage of partial two-way learning over one-way learning is that the student and teacher are participating in the process at the same time. This means that the teacher can receive information from the student on any points that need clarification during the learning experience. Another advantage of partial two-way learning is that it can reach very large groups of students at the same time if satellite transmission is used. The footprint of many of the satellites used for educational purposes covers the entire North American continent.

The disadvantages of partial two-way learning formats are related to the type of transmission utilized. For satellite-based systems, installation and transmission costs can be a major drawback. An earth station uplink can cost between $500,000 to $1,000,000 to buy and install. Transmission costs are about $500 to $650 per hour, depending upon the time of use and the transmission band utilized. Scheduling for classes can be difficult in that there are a limited number of satellites in orbit and these must be scheduled.

Production for satellite transmissions requires a number of technical experts that may not be available on the usual college campus. Most students are used to seeing high quality productions, such as those seen on the evening national news, and this level of production requires scripting, production, and a number of other costly activities. Aircraft radar and weather interference from thunderstorms can disrupt satellite transmissions. These forms of interference vary with the transmission band used. The major disadvantage of the microwave transmission format is that reception is limited to only those locations that have receiving sites. The costs of installing and maintaining transmission towers can be very expensive. Thunderstorms can also disrupt transmission on microwave systems.

Full two-way learning adds the major advantage of real time student-to-teacher interaction. This format has the same advantages of partial two-way learning, but at twice the cost. An exception is the use of compressed video technology. This approach has the advantage of lower start-up costs—about $60,000 per unit installed. Since this technology is relatively new, start-up costs will likely decrease in the next few years when more venders move into the market. When existing phone lines are used for the transmissions, operation costs are lower. Compressed video is easy to use by people without technical training, such as teachers and students. There is real time visual, audio, slides, fax, and taping capabilities in most compressed video systems.

A disadvantage of compressed video is that the equipment is highly sophisticated and sensitive. The ease with which the compressed video equipment can be used, even its appearance, often makes users think that they are handling home television and video equipment. Improper use of compressed video equipment can lead to transmission failures (e.g., hard disk crash or failure of the software to boot).

THE UNIVERSITY OF TENNESSEE, MEMPHIS EXPERIENCE

The University of Tennessee Memphis College of Nursing has used all of the forms of telecommunication described here with the exception of microwave transmission. Almost every potential problem that can be expected has occurred as well. We used the electronic telephone bridge equipment to connect several sites in rural Tennessee with on-going classes in Memphis. The faculty had trouble getting the handout and visual materials to all of the students on time; mail service was not always reliable. Sometimes during a class, one or more of the sites would be disconnected requiring a redial. We enjoyed using the satellite system until our first bills arrived. Quickly, we learned that we could not afford this system for only a few students. We also learned that faculty were not good at television production, although, the costly staff in the studio were excellent.

Today, we are using compressed interactive video equipment to outreach our Master of Science in Nursing (MSN) program to one distant site in the state. So far, 33 students have obtained their MSN degrees by using telecommunication distant learning, and an additional 20 are currently enrolled. All courses in our MSN program, didactic and clinical, are provided over the system. Meetings can take place at any time between students and teachers or between students for seminars, conferences, advisement, thesis work, or any other type of usual interaction. Each end of the system consists of a built-in PC AT compatible microcomputer, full duplex audio, an in-band fax exchange, Pen Pal Graphics interactive annotation capability, and the ability to capture and store video or computer images to the hard disk for later retrieval and forwarding. The system has a port to videotape classes for students who are unable to attend.

We are currently using two 56K AT&T® lines between the two sites. This is equivalent to 27 regular phone lines. These lines are leased and are not charged by the use. We pay about $11,000 per year for them. The system has three cameras per site: (1) one camera has zoom and full range of motion from a TV type changer, (2) one camera is fixed, we aim it at a board, and (3) one camera is used for overheads and slides. The teacher can change cameras at either site from the hand held changer.

The 56K AT&T® lines we use are a little slow in transmission, resulting in slight waterfalls if there is rapid movement. Our lines are being upgraded to a T1 which will greatly improve the picture. New compression software is being installed also. Thus, we will only need about one fourth of the T1 capability to maintain acceptable levels of transmission. Additional sites are being developed in rural Tennessee. This will require the use of a switching device to accommodate multiple sites. We will also be providing our RN and MSN programs over the system within the next year.

Through the use of distant learning technology, the faculty of the University of Tennessee Memphis College of Nursing are able to bring advanced education to many rural locations. This approach is different from traditional satellite education in that our students in rural locations can make use of the entire faculty, staff, and other students for their learning experiences. Compressed video transmissions bring the students to the campus electronically rather than requiring that they commute up to six hours one way to attend one class. We can now move voice, images, and data over this electronic highway rather than moving students over conventional highways.

14

Distance Education: Turf and Technology

Thelma Cleveland

Nursing education programs located in the eastern part of the state of Washington have been challenged to make their programs accessible to students. Eastern Washington includes two-thirds of the geographic area of the state between the Cascade Mountains on the west and Idaho on the east. The city of Spokane, close to the Idaho border, is the "hub" of eastern Washington and the Inland Northwest, and is the largest metropolitan area between Seattle and Minneapolis-St. Paul. The remainder of this region is primarily rural, with medium to small-sized communities located throughout.

Two baccalaureate and higher degree nursing programs in Spokane have been particularly active in addressing the matter of accessibility in eastern Washington: The Intercollegiate Center for Nursing Education (ICNE) and the Department of Nursing at Gonzaga University. The remainder of this paper describes their approaches to providing distance education.

The Intercollegiate Center for Nursing Education is the college of nursing for a consortium composed of Eastern Washington University, Washington State University, and Whitworth College. Washington State University, a land grant, research university, serves as the Coordinating Institution for the consortium. This relationship with a land grant university influenced the ICNE to begin providing its baccalaureate program in communities outside Spokane in the mid-seventies. The ICNE currently offers two baccalaureate degree options—one for students initiating the study of nursing and one for registered nurses—as well as a master's degree program.

In the seventies, ICNE faculty traveled 150 to 205 miles each week to outreach sites in Wenatchee, Yakima, Tri-Cities (Richland, Kennewick, Pasco) and Walla Walla to teach upper division nursing courses leading to the Bachelor of Science in Nursing degree. Lower division prerequisite courses and general education courses were available at community colleges located in these cities. A number of nurses in each area completed their degrees through this program. However, as a result of budget cuts during 1980-81, the outreach program had to be discontinued. The nursing faculty, although committed to the outreach program, found weekly travel to these sites to be tiring, time consuming, and a strain on their families.

Since its beginning, the ICNE has had a strong Continuing Nursing Education Program serving eastern Washington and the Inland Northwest. Continuing education workshops, conferences, and courses have been offered regularly at approximately 15 sites throughout the region. When a new ICNE building was constructed and occupied in 1980, faculty had access to a sophisticated television production studio and media staff. The CE Program took advantage of these resources and began producing videotape nursing courses which have been aired over cable and public television, as well as through satellite television systems. Most recently, VCR home study nursing courses have been produced and made available to nurses throughout the region.

In 1981, the ICNE established a small extended campus in Yakima (200 miles southwest of Spokane), through which it offered the upper division nursing courses for the BSN degree to basic and registered nurse students. Didactic coursework is provided by ICNE-Spokane faculty through videotaped classroom presentations sent weekly to the Yakima campus. These videotaped presentations are supplemented through telephone conferences and periodic faculty travel from Spokane to Yakima. Clinical practicum courses are taught by ICNE-Yakima resident faculty. The Yakima building contains classrooms; a core library collection; small audiovisual, computer, and nursing practice laboratories; faculty offices; secretarial space; and a small student/faculty lounge. Faculty teaching videotaped courses are oriented to this medium prior to their first classes, and supportive information is provided in the ICNE Faculty Manual.

In 1990, the ICNE building in Spokane was equipped with an electronic classroom which became part of the Washington Higher Education Telecommunication System (WHETS) originating at the Washington State University (WSU) main campus in Pullman. WHETS serves WSU's branch campuses in Vancouver, Tri-Cities, and Spokane. It also is connected to the University of Washington in Seattle and to the University of Idaho in Moscow.

WHETS currently is a microwave system that provides interactive audiovisual capabilities, as well as data transmission. Line-of-site towers provide transmission between campuses. Plans have been made to extend WHETS to additional sites along the Interstate 5 Freeway in western Washington, and to Wenatchee in eastern Washington. New sites may be connected by means of fiberoptic systems.

Through WHETS, ICNE faculty may teach a cohort of students in the specially equipped classroom at the originating site while simultaneously teaching groups of students in electronic classrooms at other connected campuses. Students and faculty at all sites can see, hear, and interact with one another with assistance of media technicians located at the various campuses. The faculty member sees only one site at a time, but sites can be quickly changed from one to another to correspond with student questions and discussion. Individual faculty/students, groups of students, or a whole classroom of students may be seen and heard through the television monitors at any given point in time.

The WHETS classroom at the ICNE in Spokane contains nine monitors. Four small monitors are located on a specially designed podium with each showing a different picture: current outgoing, incoming, overhead, and the next outgoing picture. Three larger monitors are mounted at the back of the classroom in full view of the faculty member at the podium, while the last two large monitors are placed in the front of the classroom facing the students above and behind the teacher. Television cameras are located at strategic spots throughout the room, including one directly over the podium, and microphones are suspended from the ceiling. Regular tablet-arm classroom chairs are provided in the room. It takes about 30 minutes for the media personnel to get all sites on the system before classes are taught. Special panels in the ICNE's television studio control room are used to run the system.

Faculty teaching through WHETS find that they must adapt their teaching styles to accommodate this medium. They participate in comprehensive orientation practice sessions prior to teaching their first courses. In addition, they are given a WHETS handbook that addresses how to teach over WHETS. Faculty are provided continuing technical and staff support, as well as academic, administrative, and other instructional support services. Videotapes, films, slides, transparencies, pictures from books and periodicals, graphics, blackboards—almost any audiovisual instructional tool—may be used by faculty teaching over WHETS. Close-up pictures may be shown. When written material is presented on the monitors, the media technician at the control panel can insert a live picture of the instructor in a corner of the screen.

In addition to offering classes from Spokane through WHETS, the ICNE hires resident faculty on the extended campuses. These faculty may originate classes through WHETS; however, they primarily teach clinical practicum courses. As members of the ICNE faculty, every effort is made to coordinate their work with that of the Spokane faculty. They participate in course and general faculty meetings. There are frequent telephone conversations, as well as FAX and computer communications. Periodically, faculty travel between Spokane and the extended campuses. All of the instructional support services for the various courses are provided on site.

The Department of Nursing at Gonzaga University uses a somewhat different approach to distance education than the ICNE. Theirs is a blend of distance and on-campus experiences. They initiated their distance learning program in 1987, offering their baccalaureate nursing degree program part-time to registered nurses located more than 30 miles from Spokane. They expect to offer their Master of Nursing degree program as a distance education option soon. As with the ICNE programs, the same curricula are taught at distance sites as are taught at the main nursing campus. The distance education programs are based on adult learning principles.

Gonzaga's Nursing Department sends videotaped classes to the students for home study. Both nursing and non-nursing courses, except the physical and biological sciences, are prepared for home study. Non-nursing courses include such offerings as philosophy, religion, social sciences, literature, and statistics. Students who do not have sufficient physical and biological credits from their previous nursing program to meet the baccalaureate requirements may take courses at a nearby college or may take challenge examinations through Gonzaga University.

Arrangements for clinical practica are made within a 50-mile radius of where the students live. Masters-prepared adjunct faculty are hired from the area to teach the clinical practicum courses. They travel to the Spokane campus for orientation and for periodic meetings. Conversely, Spokane faculty go periodically to the distance clinical sites and meet with agency personnel, the adjunct faculty and the students. At least three times a semester, students travel to the Gonzaga University campus in Spokane and attend classes with the nursing students enrolled there. They also meet with the Spokane faculty during these visits.

Students enrolled in Gonzaga University's distance education baccalaureate nursing program live throughout the state of Washington, in Montana, Alaska, and British Columbia, Canada. One student enrolled in the program was transferred by the military to Ohio and completed the program from there.

Schools of nursing that offer distance education opportunities have a number of issues to address to ensure quality programs. These include (1) developing procedures to assure that course materials are distributed to the off-campus students; (2) obtaining permission to incorporate copyrighted audiovisual materials into videotaped or transmitted offerings; (3) making arrangements for proctoring examinations at all sites; (4) providing support resources, such as library services and materials, computers and computer software, audiovisual hardware and software, and nursing supplies; (5) developing communication linkages through low-cost telephone systems, FAX, and computers; (6) accessing the distance education technology and technical linkages; and (7) implementing formative and summative evaluations of the courses and of the technology used to teach them.

Community building, communication, and coordination also are essential to the success of distance education endeavors. This must occur between faculty and support staff, faculty and students, among administrators and staff, and between the main campus and the off-campus sites. Complex logistics are involved and must be addressed.

The shortage of well-prepared nurses, the increasing number of older students, and the reality of place-bound persons seeking a career in nursing or advancement in the profession demand new approaches to education. Distance education is one approach to solving the problem of access. While there are disadvantages to this approach, such as faculty time and workload issues, capital and operating costs, and limited class interaction if mostly videotaped presentations are provided, both the ICNE and Gonzaga University have found that quality programs can be offered through distance learning technology coupled with in-person faculty teaching of clinical practicum courses.

PART SIX

Alternative Nursing Practice

15

Case Management: Within and Beyond the Walls

Helen R. Connors

In 1983, the University of Kansas School of Nursing received a federally funded grant to develop and implement a continuing education program designed to increase the statewide distribution of nurses prepared to perform case management. The Nursing Assessment and Management of the Frail Elderly (NAMFE) program was designed to increase nurses' knowledge and skills necessary to assess health status and manage care for frail elderly in a manner which would optimize self-care capabilities and promote efficient use of existing support resources.

The program consists of eight learning modules which focus on developing a systematic approach to the comprehensive functional assessment and care coordination of frail elderly residing in the community. Skills emphasized in the program include: (1) comprehensive assessment of the client's physical, social, psychological, and environmental status to determine level of functional ability; (2) assessment of availability and adequacy of informal and formal support resources; (3) linking the client to appropriate resources and monitoring the effectiveness of these resources; (4) self-care education, advocacy, and support for caregivers; and (5) evaluation of outcomes of care.

The conceptual framework for the curriculum is derived from nursing process, case management, and self-care theory. The stages of the nursing process were merged with the role and functions of the case manager in order to provide the framework for nursing case management. The concepts of Orem's self-care model were integrated throughout the curriculum to maximize the self-care potential of the individual and family. The course was approved for 64 contact hours of continuing education credit or for 3 hours of undergraduate or graduate credit. A variety of teaching strategies, which incorporate adult learning principles, were used for both the didactic and clinical components.

To evaluate the goals and objectives of NAMFE, it was necessary to develop instruments that assessed nurse participants' knowledge and skills of case management. Pre- and posttests were developed for each module to assess participants' cognitive abilities. In addition, the Competency Behaviors of the Case Manager Inventory (CBCMI) was developed to assess nurses' perceived ability to perform the required clinical behaviors associated with case management and the perceived importance of these behaviors to clinical practice (Connors, 1989).

The program was taught in 16 sites throughout the state of Kansas and at one site in Iowa and Oklahoma, respectively. When the grant which supported the development of this program ended in June 1988, 272 nurses from 66 counties in Kansas and bordering states had completed the course.

PURPOSE OF STUDY

The purpose of this study was to assess the impact of the program on the practice of nurses. The following research questions were addressed: (1) Is there a significant difference in the self-reported frequency of use of case management skills between nurses who have completed the NAMFE program (NAMFE group) and nurses who have not (comparison group)? (2) Is there a significant difference between the self-reported frequency of use of these skills among the three types of practice settings (community health, hospital, and nursing home for the NAMFE group)? (3) What are the perceived, self-reported, deterrents to the use of case management skills?

METHODOLOGY

A quasi-experimental controlled study, with a posttest only design, was used. The sample consisted of two groups, the NAMFE group and the comparison group. The NAMFE group was comprised of 65 nurses who completed the NAMFE program on or before May, 1987, and who were willing to participate in this study. The comparison group was composed of 57 nurses whose backgrounds were similar to the NAMFE group. Although, these nurses were enrolled in the NAMFE program, they had not participated in any of the course work.

Data for the study were gathered from two self-reported questionnaires: the Competency Behaviors of the Case Manager Inventory (CBCMI) and the Demographic/Biographic Questionnaire (D/BQ).

For the comparison group, these data were part of routine information gathered on all students in the NAMFE program during their orientation and were used for program evaluation. For the NAMFE group, data were collected by a mailed survey.

The CBCMI was developed prior to this study as part of the NAMFE program. Nursing process and case management provided the major theoretical positions from which the competency inventory was developed. The specific tasks of the case manager, as described by Austin (1983) and Steinberg and Carter (1983), were grouped into the organizing framework of nursing process/case management. This process produced six dimensions: (1) entry, (2) assessment, (3) nursing diagnosis, (4) goal setting and service care planning, (5) implementation, and (6) evaluation. Each dimension contained a list of specific behaviors totaling 68 items in all. A five-point Likert-type scale provided the measurement design for this instrument to assess self-perceived importance and adequacy of preparation for performance of the specified behaviors. For the purpose of this study, an additional scale was added to the data collection instrument in order to determine the frequency with which the participants used case management skills in their current nursing practice. The revised instrument was used by the NAMFE faculty (Fall, 1987 and Spring, 1988) to obtain prelearning data from new NAMFE students (comparison group) during orientation to the course. The same instrument was used to query NAMFE graduates (NAMFE group). In addition, NAMFE graduates were asked to identify deterrents to the use of case management skills in their practice.

RESULTS AND DISCUSSION

In order to assess similarities between the NAMFE and comparison groups, items on the D/BQ were examined. Age, educational level, place of employment, and type of position were similar for both groups (see Tables 1, 2, 3, and 4). Staff nurses and nurses employed by hospitals comprised the largest group of participants in this study; nevertheless, nursing home nurses and community health nurses provided the next largest groups. This suggests that case management for the elderly is an important facet of care across all health care settings. It also helps confirm the hypothesis that the job market requires nurses to perform these skills regardless of their preparation or practice arena.

Next, scores derived from the CBCMI use scale were analyzed to determine differences in the self-reported use of case management skills between the two groups. A frequency distribution of the use scale, skill by skill, was calculated and totaled. The NAMFE group's reported use of the CBCMI skills was 73 percent, whereas the comparison group

Table 1
Age

Variable	NAMFE Group f n=65	%	Comparison Group f n=57	%
Age				
20–29 years	2	3.0	5	8.7
30–39 years	22	33.8	23	40.3
40–49 years	20	30.7	17	29.8
50–59 years	17	26.2	11	19.3
60–69 years	4	6.1	1	1.8

Table 2
Education Level

Variable	NAMFE Group f n=65	%	Comparison Group f n=57	%
Education: Highest level in nursing				
Associate Degree	11	16.7	12	21.1
Diploma	29	43.9	23	38.5
BSN	19	28.8	20	35.0
Masters	7	10.6	2	3.5
Education: Highest non-nursing degree				
Associate Degree	3	13.6	4	21.0
Baccalaureate	12	54.5	9	47.4
Masters	6	27.3	6	31.5
Doctorate	1	4.5	0	0

Table 3
Place of Employment

Variable	NAMFE Group f n=65	%	Comparison Group f n=57	%
Place of employment				
Community health	14	21.5	15	26.3
Office	2	3.1	1	1.7
School of nursing	2	3.1	2	3.5
Social agency or SRS	3	4.6	4	7.0
Nursing home	17	26.2	12	21.0
Hospital	21	32.3	17	29.8
Other	7	10.7	6	10.5

Table 4
Type of Position

Variable	NAMFE Group f n=65	%	Comparison Group f n=57	%
Type of position				
Administrator	6	9.2	6	10.5
Inservice or staff dv.	1	1.5	1	1.8
Supervisor or asst.	9	13.8	11	19.3
Head nurse or asst.	7	10.8	6	10.5
Case manager	9	13.8	5	8.8
Staff	20	30.8	14	24.6
Educator	3	4.6	5	8.8
CNS or nurse pract.	0	0.0	1	1.8
Quality ass. or IPR	4	6.2	1	1.8
Other	6	9.2	7	12.3

reported a 68 percent use of these skills. A chi square analysis showed no significant difference in the overall frequency of use of these skills between the two groups.

For the NAMFE group, a one-way analysis of variance (ANOVA) was performed to determine significant differences between the self-reported frequency of use of case management skills and the type of practice setting (i.e., community health, hospital, nursing home) of the nurses. Again, results were not significant.

Results of these analyses suggest that in today's health care environment, case management skills are being utilized in a wide range of practice settings; they are not specific to the traditional community-based nursing environment. The need for these skills in the various practice settings also was evident from the demographic data since participants about to enter the NAMFE program (comparison group) were distributed almost equally between the three major practice sites: (1) community health (26 percent), (2) nursing home (21 percent), and, (3) hospital (30 percent). The demand for these skills in current clinical practice was illustrated further by the fact that on the D/BQ 68 percent of the comparison group stated that they were using case management skills in their clinical practice. Yet, 78 percent reported that these skills were not taught in their basic nursing program and 79 percent reported that they had not participated in a continuing education program designed to teach these skills. All subjects who reported having had some of these skills in their basic nursing program stated that the content was integrated throughout the curriculum; none had participated in a specific course designed to teach case management skills. It also was of interest to note that although there was no significant difference in the use of these skills between the two groups, NAMFE versus comparison, 92 percent of the NAMFE group indicated that the NAMFE course had a positive effect on their approach to patient care. The exact nature of this positive effect was not assessed in this study.

Because the results of this study demonstrated no significant difference in the use of case management skills between the NAMFE group and the comparison group and no significant difference in the use of case management skills among practice settings for the NAMFE group, it was further hypothesized that perhaps the job market was requiring nurses to use these skills when, in fact, nurses were not adequately prepared to do so. Data from the adequacy of preparation for performance scale of the CBCMI were analyzed to address this new research question. A Student's t test for independent groups was utilized to determine significant differences in the self-reported adequacy of preparation for performance of case management skills between the NAMFE and the comparison groups. Analysis revealed a significant difference at the $p < .0001$ level.

These results suggest that although nurses in a variety of settings are required to perform case management skills, they do not consider themselves prepared to do so. For this reason, they were seeking a continuing education program designed to increase their knowledge and skill base. As a result of this continuing education experience, they perceived themselves to be better prepared to perform their job functions. They also believed that this education had a positive effect on their approach to patient care. As Patton (1986) has suggested, underutilization or nonutilization of skills taught through continuing education may be attributed to too narrow a definition of utilization. Patton has proposed that evaluation be viewed in terms of instrumental and conceptual use. Instrumental use refers to concrete actions; conceptual use gives credit to how the participant thinks about or evaluates the action. In other words, although continuing education may not change the way nurses practice (instrumental use), it may change the way they think about their practice (conceptual use). Thus, it prepares them better to function in today's rapidly changing health care environment.

When the NAMFE group was asked about the deterrents to the use of case management skills, insufficient time and lack of support from nursing administrators or supervisors accounted for 62 percent of the perceived deterrents. These deterrents suggest the need to reevaluate the skills in view of the practice settings and to educate administrators and managers regarding the importance of these skills and their impact on health care delivery.

SUMMARY AND CONCLUSION

Results of this study demonstrated no significant differences in the frequency of the instrumental use of case management skills between nurses who graduated from the NAMFE program (NAMFE group) and those who were about to enter the program (comparison group); however, there was a significant difference ($p < .0001$ level) in the perceived preparation for performance of these skills between the two groups. Currently, few educational programs provide nurses with the essential knowledge and skills to function in the role of case manager; yet, the job market demands it of them. The program was able to fill the gap between education and service.

Although the NAMFE course no longer is available for continuing education credit through the University of Kansas School of Nursing, the course currently is offered as an elective for senior level students and graduate students. Also, the curriculum materials and teaching strategies manuals, developed as part of this grant, and consultations regarding the use of these materials are available.

Table 5
Student t Test Showing Differences in
Perceived Preparation for Performance

	n	x	sd	t	p
Dimensions					
Entry					
NAMFE	65	31.6	5.4	2.8	.0056
Comparison	57	28.3	7.4		
Assessment					
NAMFE	65	67.2	12.3	4.9	.0001
Comparison	57	55.9	13.0		
Nursing diagnosis					
NAMFE	65	14.7	3.1	4.6	.0001
Comparison	57	12.1	3.2		
Service care planning					
NAMFE	65	49.2	11.5	5.1	.0001
Comparison	57	38.9	10.3		
Implementation					
NAMFE	65	48.8	11.9	3.6	.0001
Comparison	57	39.2	12.3		
Evaluation					
NAMFE	65	29.8	7.6	3.6	.0005
Comparison	57	24.6	8.4		
TOTAL					
NAMFE	65	241.3	46.5	4.82	.0001
Comparison	57	198.9	49.4		

REFERENCES

Austin, C. D. (1983). Case management in long-term care: Options and opportunities. *Health and Social Work* (Reprint No. 0360–7283/83).

Connors, H. R. (1989). Impact evaluation of a statewide continuing education program. *Journal of Continuing Education in Nursing, 20*(2), 64–69.

Patton, M. Q. (1986). *Utilization-focused evaluation.* Beverly Hills: Sage.

Steinberg, R. M., & Carter, G. W. (1983). *Case management and the elderly.* Lexington, MA: Lexington.

16

A Caring Community within Acute-Care Institutions? It Can Be Done, and Here's How

Eloise M. Balasco

At Mercy Hospital in Portland, Maine, we have implemented a clinical promotion program designed to recognize and reward the development of practical knowledge, moral agency, and discretionary judgment and caring within the practice of nurses. This program uses Benner's (1984) work as a framework to identify the qualitative distinctions within the changing nursing practice (Balasco & Black, 1988).

Our program is built on two premises. First, nurses providing direct care to patients and families implement the primary and central mission of the nursing profession. Second, clinical practice is a worthwhile endeavor to be supported by all other roles in the nursing organization. Within the structure of primary nursing, the clinical nurse is accountable for the continuous relationship with primary patients and families. It is in this relationship that the unique human concerns of the patient and family are expressed, listened to, and addressed (Balasco, 1990).

Caring is the foundation of the practice of nursing as well as its moral imperative. Thus, the description of a highly competent practice of nursing must make explicit the relationship between advanced clinical knowledge and judgment and highly evolved caring practices. The caring relationship between a patient and nurse is the common denominator in all stories about making a difference (Benner, 1988).

To understand the unique and central place of caring in the nursing practice, it is important to distinguish between disease and illness. The treatment of disease is the primary focus of the practice of medicine. The physician relies upon scientific principles which explain how organ dysfunction manifests itself in a way that is generalizable from one person to the next. Illness, on the other hand, is the patient's particular response to disease; it is the human experience of loss or dysfunction. Knowledge about a specific person in a particular situation is involved in the understanding of illness. The illness discourse tells of the fear and frustration of being inside a body that is breaking down. The treatment of illness is the primary focus of the practice of nursing. The human concerns of the patient and family, expressed in a relationship characterized by involvement and concern, determine the strategic approach of the nurse. The nurse's ability to participate in the experience of illness with the patient encourages the authentic expression of feeling and need, empowering the patients to achieve maximum control over their recovery. The caring relationship between patient and nurse facilitates genuine healing as well as cure (Benner & Wrubel, 1989; Frank, 1981; Niziolek & Hall, 1990).

Because theoretical knowledge held by the nurse is nursing only when applied to the particular situation of the individual in need of care, the essence of the nursing practice is best captured by the study of practical activity—what nurses do when they are engaged in everyday situations with patients and families (Pellegrino, 1989). Hermeneutic phenomenology is one method allowing for the interpretation of lived experience. It captures most adequately the meanings of everyday practical activity: telling the story is the most effective way to illuminate the practical knowledge, judgment, and moral agency involved in caring practices by highly competent nurses (Wilson & Hutchinson, 1991).

Therefore, the clinical narrative has become the cornerstone of our promotion program at Mercy Hospital. Narrative uncovers meanings and feelings in the relationships between nurses and patients. In that respect, narrative is quite distinct from case study, which highlights the issue and reports only the facts. Narrative discloses and preserves the concerns, fears, hopes, conversations, and issues between patient and nurse (Benner, 1991). With the use of the narrative, the nurse establishes ownership and accountability for practice; so, the narrative contributes to the development of a professional practice model (Tappan & Brown, 1989). Narrative also discloses where and how the vision and values of the nursing profession are experienced in the practice. In addition, narrative is a powerful tool with which to chart clinical knowledge development: it makes clear the qualitative distinctions of the different stages of the nursing practice.

When nurses wish to seek promotion to advanced levels of practice at Mercy Hospital, they are asked to prepare a portfolio which includes two practice narratives or exemplars. Nurses present their portfolio to the board of review of the clinical promotion program. This peer review process supports our belief that nursing is a practice, located within a complex social, historical, and cultural tradition of caring attitudes, skills, and practices. Moreover, this context cannot be fully understood or appreciated by persons outside the tradition (Balasco & Cathcart, 1992).

The following exemplar was presented by Beverly Bridges, RN, a nurse in the PostAnesthesia Care Unit (PACU), in the process of her promotion to Clinical Nurse II:

DONNA'S STORY

Donna was a 38-year-old woman with a past history of breast cancer. She had undergone surgery in another state. She and her present surgeon were not pleased with the appearance of her breasts after the plastic surgery. Today her surgery was more extensive breast reconstruction involving a long surgical course. She had been well cared for in the PACU by a fellow nurse whose shift was ending. As I listened to the report, I realized that Donna was probably going to be very anxious because of her history of cancer, her age, and her first unsatisfactory surgery. My plan was to be calm and reassuring through the use of my voice and physical touch.

Her eyes were wide open and I introduced myself to her and explained everything as I did it. When I touched her hands while talking to her, I remarked to her that her hands felt cold. "They always are," she said. I offered to give her plastic gloves filled with warm water to hold and she agreed. I asked her if she wanted her husband to come and sit with her during her PACU stay. This would probably allay Mr. T's anxiety and help calm Donna by having her husband near.

Donna's anesthesiologist had ordered a postop hematocrit and hemoglobin. Today's extensive surgery had resulted in a high blood loss. Her H & H results were low: 9.3 and 26.9, relative to her normal 11 and 32 preop. Her blood pressure was low—80 to 90 systolic, compared with her normal of 120/60. I reported these levels to her surgeon who ordered two units of blood to be transfused. When I explained to Donna the need for blood replacement, she became very anxious saying she was afraid of AIDS and did not want to receive blood. I calmly explained to her the safety of receiving blood and the process of blood testing to assure the safety of transfusions. I did not want to override her rights. I felt the dilemma of preserving and protecting her right to determine her own care versus my knowledge of her body's need for blood replacement. I did not want to force any treatment on Donna without her full consent. I called her doctor to let him know her fears and her refusal. I had hoped he might want to try other methods to expand her fluid volume. "Try to convince her, she really needs the blood" he said and hung up the phone. Still mindful of her rights, yet knowing her body's need for blood, I again talked with Donna and her husband.

I then decided that I had gone as far as I could to try to convince Donna. I could see the need for another course of action to therapeutically manipulate the situation for the best outcome. I asked Donna and her husband if they would feel better talking directly to the surgeon. They readily agreed. I called Dr. W. back and told him I was putting Mr. and Mrs. T on the phone to talk with him. (I was not giving him a choice!) I wheeled Donna in her stretcher to the phone while her husband spoke on the other line. After a few questions to her doctor, Donna agreed to receive the blood and seemed comfortable with her decision.

I felt that I had respected Donna's wishes by not just giving the transfusion, "Because the doctor ordered it." Her rights had been preserved and her anxiety decreased. She had been able to take an active role in the decision-making process for her own plan of care.

I recently cared for Donna again in the PACU, after more reconstructive breast surgery. After I introduced myself, Donna looked at me and said, "I remember you. You took care of me before and gave me gloves of warm water for my hands." I wondered if her perception of her last PACU experience had been negative. I asked her, "Do you remember talking with the doctor on the phone when he explained why you needed a blood transfusion?" "No, just the gloves" she replied. I felt relieved and glad that what remained foremost in her mind was my sense of touch and concern rather than my attempt at convincing her of the safety of the blood transfusions. Her statement reaffirmed my belief that connecting with my patients, by showing concern and respect for their needs, is often more important to them than the critical procedures or treatments that I perform during the immediate postoperative event.

This narrative is an ethical discourse because it depicts a clinical situation in which Beverly Bridges reaffirmed a belief about the inherent good in her practice. Her story tells how that good was lived out in the relatively short time she spent with Donna and her husband. She is also reminded of what it means to be a nurse and of the significance and worth of her work. In that way, this narrative serves to sustain the practice (Benner, 1991).

We can assume that concrete past situations with particular patients offered Beverly Bridges memories that allowed her to anticipate Donna's needs. She develops a picture of how she might find her patient. She maps out the way in which she will approach Donna, and in doing so, presents a beautiful picture of skilled ethical comportment. Her plan to comfort and calm Donna encompasses the nuances of touch and the use of her voice. Beverly Bridges' caring practices quickly come into play; the time Donna will spend in the PACU will be short.

This narrative also illustrates the growth and development of the practice. Traditionally, PACU nursing has been focused on ensuring safe emergence from anesthesia. Previously, the episodic nature of the experience was thought to preclude a more meaningful interaction between the patient and the nurse (Allen & Swett, 1990). Beverly Bridges shows that this is not so, and in fact, her story reinforces the importance of her caring practices. She offers a rich example of how to preserve Donna's dignity and sense of person by acknowledging Donna's right to determine her own care. Beverly Bridges could have described Donna's refusal of the blood transfusion as a life threatening situation putting Donna in the position of having to make a decision between two poor choices. Instead, Beverly Bridges takes time to therapeutically manipulate the situation; thus, preserving Donna's sense of control. Beverly Bridges' moral agency comes into play as she calls the surgeon again and does not give him a choice except to do what would be helpful to her patient.

Narrative is not the only method for evaluating candidates for clinical promotion. We consider the nurse's past performance, references from colleagues and patients about the nurse's practice, and the recommendation of the nurse manager. But as Beverly Bridges' story of her care of Donna illustrates, narrative can capture, and make public, qualitative aspects of a nurse's interaction with patients, families, and physicians that reveal the rich mix of practical knowledge, judgment, caring, and moral agency constituting expert nursing practice.

REFERENCES

Allen, D., & Swett, D. L. (1990). Blending expert knowledge and caring. *Journal of Professional Nursing, 6*(4).

Balasco, E. (1990). The nurse in relationship. *Journal of Professional Nursing, 6*(1).

Balasco, E., & Black, A. (1988). Advancing nursing practice: Description, recognition and reward. *Nursing Administration Quarterly, 12*(2).

Balasco, E., & Cathcart, T. (1992). Why cross-training won't work. *Journal of Professional Nursing, 8*(2).

Benner, P. (1984). *From novice to expert: Excellence and power in clinical nursing practice.* Menlo Park, CA: Addison-Wesley.

Benner, P. (1988). Nursing as a caring profession. (Working Paper). Kansas City: American Academy of Nursing.

Benner, P. (1991). The role of experience, narrative and community in skilled ethical comportment. *Advances in Nursing Science, 14*(2).

Benner, P., & Wrubel, J. (1989). *The primacy of caring.* Menlo Park, CA: Addison-Wesley.

Frank, A. (1990). *At the will of the body: Reflections on illness.* Boston: Houghton-Mifflin.

Niziolek, C., & Hall, J. (1990). Uncovering the experts. *Journal of Professional Nursing, 6*(2).

Pellegrino, E. (1989). Theory and practice of virtue. Paper presented at the Intensive Bioethics Conference, Georgetown University, Washington, DC.

Tappan, M., & Brown, L. M. (1989). Stories told and lessons learned: Toward a narrative approach to moral development and moral education. *Harvard Educational Review, 59*(2).

Wilson, H. S., & Hutchinson, S. A. (1991). Triangulation of qualitative methods; Heideggerian hermeneutics and grounded theory. *Qualitative Health Research, 1*(2).

17

Violence Against Women: Clinical Issues

Josephine Ryan and Christine King

As many as 30 percent of all women in the United States experience physical abuse from their husbands or partners at least once in their life time. Studies suggest that each year between 2 and 4 million women are physically battered by partners including husbands, former husbands, boyfriends, and lovers. It is also known that more than one million women seek medical assistance for injuries caused by battering each year. It is known that violence and abuse experienced by women who are in relationships result in physical and emotional health problems, severely compromising a woman's ability to participate in health promotion or health maintenance activities (Kerouac, Taggart, Lescop, & Fortin, 1986).

Violence and abuse directed against women by male partners has been labeled a health care problem in disguise (Drake, 1972). Studies of women who have lived in abusive situations indicate that abused women have greater health problems than women who are not abused. Health problems include: physical injuries, miscarriages, rape, chronic pain, stress and anxiety disorders, hypertension, hyperventilation, allergic reactions, anorexia, insomnia, depression, suicide attempts, and disturbed parent-child relationships (Finkelhor & Yllo, 1983; Kerouac et al., 1986; Lion, 1977).

In a descriptive study of 130 abused women residing in eight Montreal shelters for battered women, data were collected on women's perceptions of their health and that of their children (Kerouac et al., 1986). It was found that 50 percent of the abused women reported that their health was good to excellent in comparison to the general population. Nevertheless, when asked to list injuries, physician visits, and certain conditions, their answers indicated that these women are less healthy than nonabused women. A variety of health complaints and detrimental life habits were reported, including poor diet, smoking, and drug abuse. In addition, these women were found to be more anxious and depressed, and reported more somatic symptoms than the general population.

Not only is the health of abused women compromised, but they are also less likely to access primary health care. It is noteworthy that while abused women are most likely to enter the health care system via the emergency room, there is a widespread lack of recognition of battering by health personnel in traditional settings (Bowker & Maurer, 1987; Kirz, D., 1987; McLear & Anwar, 1989; Rounsaville & Weissman, 1977). Also for child-bearing women, the one time almost all women in the United States come in contact with health care providers is at labor and delivery of the baby. Almost every woman, from the migrant worker woman to the mayor's wife, has some contact with a nurse during prenatal care, labor and delivery, or postpartum.

Despite the overall incidence of battering and its resultant physical and emotional health problems for women, health professionals fail to identify abused women. In addition, health professionals use derogatory labeling and are generally seen as judgmental and insensitive (Drake, 1982; Goldberg & Tomlanovich, 1984; Nuttall, Greaves & Lent, 1985) and less effective and helpful than other help sources (Dobash & Dobash, 1978; Bowker & Maurer, 1987). Of equal importance, Goodstein and Page (1981) suggest that the quality of health care that battered women receive often determines whether they follow through with referrals to legal, social service, and health care agencies.

The most asked question about abuse of women is, "Why do women stay?" Behind this question is the assumption that the abuse cannot be that terrible or else women would leave. This might even translate into a belief that because a woman has not left a violent relationship, she must not want to leave. Therefore, intervention has little value because women will not leave anyway. On a more basic level, this question can be even more pernicious if it is asked out of a belief that the violence may gratify a deep personal need. This is blaming the victim.

The reasons women do not leave abusive relationships are no different from the reasons women stay in any unpleasant or difficult relationship. Home is not unbearable all the time. Even in the most violent relationships, it is shelter. Women spend considerable time and energy thinking about and creating this environment. Their home contains all their belongings, their clothes, old photographs; it is familiar; neighbors, friends, and relatives provide pleasant moments; it is the home of their children and their children's neighborhood. Moving requires careful planning. Escaping sometimes means abandonment of all personal belongings, friends, and any modicum of security.

Economics is a significant factor for women not being able to leave. For women from all economic classes, divorce or separation brings a definite loss of economic security. Single mothers face economic insecurity and frequently fall into poverty. The statistics of the number of children from one parent households who currently live below the poverty level is shocking. Child support payments are seldom made by the partner. Adequate affordable housing does not exist, nor does good child care. Women face serious obstacles in finding employment.

In the United States, mainstream culture and religion encourage women to maintain intact families. Divorce is still not sanctioned by some religions. Single parents are strongly discriminated against subtly or overtly in schools, jobs, and recreation. Even though the nuclear family model no longer exists as the predominant family lifestyle, society still holds this social construction of the family.

The legal system makes it extremely difficult for women to leave an abusive relationship. Many judges trivialize the violence or blame women. Restraining orders and other civil protective orders are not backed up in many states by mandatory arrest upon violation. Thus, women might obtain a civil protective order only to have the abuser return and hurt them and their children, or even murder them. If they did leave, women have few places to go. They may have few relatives with whom to spend an extended period of time. They may have depleted their social support resources. The problem is compounded by the fact that few women have ever lived alone. Many women in the United States go from their parent's home to the home of their partner or from their parent's home to a shared apartment with female friends and then to marriage or a lover.

The lack of understanding we have about how difficult it is for women to leave abusive relationships fosters a further myth: women who live in abusive relationships tend to become helpless. This myth ignores all the areas in which women are powerful; these include parenting, work, friendships, and home management.

More importantly, this myth denies women a part in their own attempts at liberation and fosters the rescue fantasies of health care workers steeped in the medical model. Health care workers are vulnerable to their personal need for effectiveness or compliance with their advice. If they expect or want women to leave abusive relationships and women do not, or they leave and then return, health care workers may not be happy and will often find it difficult to counsel them again. In the absence of anyone validating women's efforts at keeping the family together, courageously managing children, women might accept their partners' derogatory appraisals.

Many women do not stay with their abusive partners. Women who have the right combination of personal, economic, and social supports have extricated themselves despite all the obstacles. The only person who can decide the relative balance of risks and benefits is the woman herself.

The more important question we need to ask is, "What are the resources a woman needs to get out of an abusive relationship?" Nurses are part of the resources women have to help them decide what to do about an abusive relationship. I would like to address ways in which nurses can be a part of the resources women can turn to if they are in an abusive relationship.

First, nurses can determine whether women who they see in their practice have been subjected to abuse. Second, nurses can intervene in the secondary prevention of abuse. Nurses in all practice settings are ideally positioned to help a woman who is in a violent relationship. That nurses do not intervene is evidence not of their lack of concern, but of their lack of knowledge about what to do and what is best for a woman.

Nurses in most educational programs and in most practice settings have not received the requisite knowledge or skills to feel comfortable in intervening with women they know or suspect may be experiencing violence. Neither do they know how to ask about violence directly. Yet, nurses are excellent interviewers, educators, and, counsellors and would intervene if they felt comfortable and assured.

Through practice with abused women, research, and interaction with advocates for women, we have come to understand that women need to be asked directly about abuse in their lives. If women are not being abused, they can learn that health care workers consider abuse an important health issue. Alternatively, this may help women when a relative or friend is abused. If women are abused, you will have decreased their guilt, shame, and isolation, factors that perhaps normalized the violence.

Letting a woman know that violence is a prevalent problem—the nurse will ask about it even if the woman does not present signs of injuries—is in itself a powerful intervention. Women who are not married may be suffering from abuse from previous partners or current lovers. Young women may be in violent dating relationships. Older women may be suffering abuse from adult children or partners. Since there is no way to rationally exclude any woman, all women should be asked.

There are several ways to ask about abuse. One is to preface questions with the statement that abuse of women is extremely common and that you ask all women these questions. Two examples are: "I ask all my women clients if they are in a relationship or have an association with a person who is abusing or attempting to control them" or "Many women in our society experience abuse from their partners; is anything like this happening in your life?" Nurses can also ask a series of screening questions preceded by a generalization (see Table 1). These screening questions, developed from research and clinical work

Table 1
Exemplary Abuse Assessment Questions

1. Do you feel emotionally abused by your partner?
2. Has your partner ever hit, slapped, kicked, or otherwise physically hurt you?
3. Are you afraid of your partner?
4. Do you feel your partner tries to control you?
5. Has your partner ever forced you into sex that you did not wish to participate in?

by the Nursing Research Consortium on Violence and Abuse, can be asked to any woman in any setting. Much depends, of course, on the caring and careful way these questions are asked. Since there is no way to assess abuse, unless there are obvious physical indicators, it is good practice to ask them to all women. They should be asked in privacy and in a caring manner. There has been some criticism from the lesbian community, that openly lesbian women are not assessed for abuse. Violence does occur in lesbian relationships as well and lesbians should be assessed. (Note that all questions should be worded in a gender free form.)

Many nurses may initially feel uncomfortable, because they view intimate relationships as too personal to ask about (King & Ryan, 1989). It is not unlike doing the first nursing assessment interview and being selective about questions you would ask and those you skipped over. Nevertheless, the realization that violence and abuse is a major health problem for women should demonstrate the importance of these questions. If the woman does disclose her abuse to you, by answering yes to any of the screening question, then you can provide advocacy. Remember, abused women are very resourceful. You are the tool to their further empowerment. Woman is the actor, you are the facilitator. Women do not wish to be rescued, only to be listened to, counselled, and presented with some referral options. Intervention does not take long, only a few moments, but it can go a long way in the secondary prevention of violence and in the promotion of health for women and their children.

Although assessing and intervening with individual women about abuse may be seen as an individually focused response to the societal problem of abuse to women, it is actually more than that. The screening questions and advocacy protocols are transferable knowledge. They can easily be taught, learned, and implemented in every setting in which women come for health care either for themselves or for their children. In addition, the discussion necessary to get the assessment and intervention implemented in your institution will be instructive for all health care workers involved.

If we can ask every woman in the United States these questions just as we examine the breasts and cervix of every woman, and if we can intervene effectively, we can be assured to have responded to C. Everett Koop, the former Surgeon General, when he named violence against women as the number one health problem for women in this country.

REFERENCES

Bowker, L. H., & Maurer, L. (1987). The medical treatment of battered wives. *Women & Health, 12*(1), 25–45.

Dobash, R. E., & Dobash, R. P. (1979). *Violence against wives.* New York: Free Press.

Drake, V. K. (1982). Battered Women: A health care problem. *Image, 19*(2), 40–47.

Finkelhor, D., & Yllo, K. (1983). License to rape: Sexual abuse of wives. *American Journal of Psychotherapy, 34,* 334–50.

Goldberg, W. G., & Tomlanovich, M. C. (1984). Domestic violence victims in the emergency department. *Journal of the American Medical Association, 251,* 3259–3264.

Goodstein, R. K., & Page, A. W. (1981). Battered wife syndrome: Overview of dynamics and treatment. *American Journal of Psychiatry, 138,* 1036–1044.

Kerouac, S., Taggart, M. E., Lescop, J., & Fortin, M. F. (1986). Dimensions of health in violent families. *Health Care for Women International, 7,* 413–426.

King, M. C., & Ryan, J. (1989). A study of the health care needs of women experiencing violence. *Proceedings of the 3rd NNVAW Conference.* Concord, CA.

Kirz, D. (1987). Emergency department responses to battered women: Resistance to medicalization. *Social Problems, 34*(1), 501–513.

Lion, J. R. (1977). Clinical aspects of wifebeating. In M. Roy (Ed.), *Battered women: A psychosocial study of domestic violence* (pp. 126–136). New York: Van Nostrand Reinhold.

McLear, S. V., & Anwar, R. (1989). A study of battered women presenting in an emergency department. *American Journal of Public Health, 79*(1), 65–66.

Nuttall, S. E., Greaves, L. J., & Lent, B. (1985). *Canadian Journal of Public Health, 76,* 297–299.

Rounsaville, B. J., & Weissman, M. M. (1977). Battered women: A medical problem requiring detection. *International Journal of Psychiatry Medicine, 8*(2), 191–202.

Rounsaville, B. J., & Weissman, M. M. (1977). Coping with domestic violence: Social support and psychological health among battered women. *American Journal of Community Psychology, 11*(6), 629–654.

PART SEVEN

Legal and Economic Challenges for the Decade

18

Home Care: The Direction of Future Health Care Services

*Cathy Frasca**

*H*ome care today is a long way from the traditional home care and visiting nurse services of the past. Home care has evolved from providing basic nursing services for the poor elderly to a full spectrum of health care and related services for people of all ages. Major influences in the growth of home care were the introduction of Medicare Home Care Reimbursement in 1965 and the implementation of both the Hospital Prospective Payment System (PPS) and Diagnostic Related Groupings (DRG) in 1984, when hospitals moved from cost reimbursement to a payment system based upon specific diagnostic-related groupings. As an outgrowth of the PPS and DRGs, acute care patients were discharged from hospitals in the more intense phase of their illness, requiring a multiplicity of products and services. These ranged from wellness programs and basic personal care and support services to specialty care and high technology treatments. These sicker patients required a full complement of qualified, experienced professionals and support staff. This growing trend reflects that the needs of these sicker patients will be even more pronounced in future years.

SHHS/HHA PROGRAM MODEL

In this chapter I describe home care today by using the South Hills Health System Home Health Agency (SHHS/HHA) as a hospital-based

---

*Edited by Helen Triebsch, Director, Research & Development SHHS/HHA.

program model. SHHS/HHA started in 1963 (two years before Medicare home care reimbursement). It was a department of Homestead Hospital, a small medical/surgical community hospital in the "Steel Valley" of Pittsburgh, Pennsylvania. The patient census of this nonprofit, hospital-based HHA soon reached 400, far surpassing the hospital inpatient capacity of less than 250 beds. Other area hospitals and their physicians soon became interested in this home care program as its reputation of excellence spread. Letters of agreement were prepared for participating hospitals to join this most unique home care program. In essence, participation afforded select HHA staff members access to the facility and patients. The agency, in turn, provided the hospitals with a full complement of readily available home care services. Over the years, the initial letters of agreement have evolved into sophisticated contracts with each participating hospital. This allows the agency to more effectively govern each of the satellite home care departments.

The agency is currently structured as a single, nonprofit, hospital-based, Medicare-certified, accredited by the Joint Commission on Accreditation of Hospitals (JCAHO), licensed HHA with 9 satellite home care departments. Each satellite home care department operates, essentially, as a home care department within each participating hospital. Even though home care staff members are home care employees and function as an extension of the HHA, they also must adhere to all policies, procedures and guidelines of each participating hospital. Each home care department has a full management staff who participate in key meetings at each hospital and have a matrix link to the hospital chief executive officer or his or her designee. The management staff reports directly to a supervisor located at the administrative offices. This close link ensures that patients referred to the home care department have no interruption in their continuum of care as they are discharged from acute care to home care or vice versa.

This HHA has grown to become the largest program of its kind in the nation, with an average daily census of about 3,000 patients, with approximately 400 professional and support staff generating close to 300,000 home visits per year.

ADVANTAGES AND DISADVANTAGES OF A HOSPITAL-BASED HOME HEALTH AGENCY

Advantages

1. HHA functions as an integral part of the hospital's system, having ready access to hospital facilities, resources and expertise to utilize for ensuring the provision of a comprehensive, coordinated continuum of high quality care. Home care intake staff act as a vital link to complement the hospital discharge planning process.

2. HHA assists the hospital in reducing the acute inpatient length of stay (LOS) by identifying and eliminating problematic DRG/LOS through home care intervention, support, and service program expansion.
3. HHA provides ambulatory care and outpatient surgical areas to patients who have not been admitted yet require skilled follow-up services.
4. HHA increases the quality of care, while decreasing potential liability to the hospital, by providing a direct link for acute care patients leaving the hospital during a more intense phase of their illness.
5. HHA acts as a feeder into all other hospital-related services (e.g., ambulatory care, emergency room, long-term care, and surgi-center).
6. HHA provides a high synergistic value in education and communication between acute care and home care providers.

Disadvantages

1. Qualified, experienced home care staff are not readily available. Community health is a specialty service not only for nurses, but also for all therapists, aides, and other caregivers, particularly now that high technology treatments are moving into the home.
2. Lack of understanding within some hospital departments regarding unique needs of HHA result in difficulty in meeting certain needs and challenges (i.e., organizational structure, personnel issues such as pay scales and on-call procedures).
3. Hospital-based home care is highly regulated and HHA requirements for certification, accreditation, and licensure are atypical of those needed for acute care. The HHA must comply as a department of the hospital while still meeting all its needs (i.e., policies relating to travel, dress code, inclement weather, and care in high risk areas).
4. Home care is essentially cost or less-than-cost reimbursed.

A BALANCE OF ADVANTAGES AND DISADVANTAGES

1. Indirect allocation of Medicare costs from hospital to home care, helping to alleviate acute care costs, may result in higher home care rates. Medicare add-on to hospital-based home care cost caps are most appropriate to meet increased costs. Nevertheless they may give hospital HHAs a cost-competitive disadvantage.

2. Liability of home care services may be an added safeguard for early discharge of hospital acute care patients, but may add potential liability to hospital-based home health agencies.

3. Expanded JCAHO accreditation survey results will impact the hospital and all related businesses including their home care program as the lowest ratings will prevail systemwide.

4. The more complex organizational structure within which the hospital-based agency must exist delays the decision-making process when timely discussions may be key to remaining service-competitive. Nevertheless, availability of resources within the hospital can facilitate agency operations.

PLANNING AND DEVELOPING A HOME HEALTH AGENCY

In order to develop a new home care program or new or expanded home care services, it is helpful to use basic planning techniques that can be applied specifically to home care. Basic planning for any type of venture has vital elements that serve as a foundation for building and developing any program or service entity. At the very least, five basic types of information are needed:

1. Assessment of the HHA's external environment.

2. Internal assessment of the HHA to include types of services provided, admission and visit volume of each service, and personnel available.

3. Analysis of patients to include payor type and diagnoses.

4. Customer-referral source analysis.

5. Competitor analysis to expand services provided and to analyze pricing issues.

PLANNING CRITERIA THAT HAVE PROVEN HELPFUL

1. *Specific volume.* Consider the number of admissions and visits projected and actually made for each service type. Also, assess visits per day and hours per visit for each home care service line. Discipline-specific productivity standards are essential. Within the admissions profile, consider diagnoses and visit intensity (i.e., visits per admission). Assess the number of reimbursable visits and develop payor mix profiles by overall volume, volume by diagnoses and visits per admission by payor or by diagnosis.

2. *Ability to meet need.* First consider current staff resources on hand and assess turnover rates from the last two to three years. Then consider how many qualified staff are available in a given area. Within the latter, assess the competition's ability to attract and maintain staff. Analyze wage and benefit packages.

3. *Costs.* Consider actual cost per unit for each service type and the aggregate unit cost per visit. This is even more critical with periodic threats of Medicare reimbursement to consider changing aggregate to discipline-specific cost reimbursement.

4. *Benefits.* Identify tangible and intangible benefits of home health services to the patient, to the agency and, if hospital-based, to the parent hospital.

5. *Patient and physician acceptability.* Consider how these two groups will accept home health services. Many physicians are starting their own HHAs and other related businesses. In addition, users' past experiences with similar services will impact attitudes toward a new business or venture.

6. *Financing.* Assess past, current, and future reimbursement trends in all service types. Consider availability of alternative funding.

7. *Return on investment.* Is the project worth what it costs in time, effort, and dollars? Consider all costs involved in maintaining the business or expanding into new services. Project revenues and calculable return on investment. Is it worth it?

8. *Operating costs.* Consider all office needs from space (new or existing) to office furniture to computer needs. If leasing, you need to exercise caution not to get locked into a costly, long-term lease that may jeopardize cost limits under a home care PPS.

As the needs of intensely ill patients increase, every effort must be made to diversify to meet those needs in the most efficient and cost effective manner. Home care, in most instances, can provide a wider scope and higher concentration of services at the lowest possible unit cost per visit. Such services demonstrate HHA's willingness and ability to meet the needs of the patient and of the referral sources in not only a more cost effective environment, but a more healing one as well. Two excellent examples are care of the ventilator patient in the home (as opposed to acute care or skilled-nursing facility setting) and providing intravenous antibiotic services to the patient who would otherwise have a lengthy acute care stay.

Controlling cost per visit is most critical during the transition from a cost reimbursed system to some future type of PPS system in home care. The SHHS/HHA has had many consultancies through the years to study its efficiencies. Most recently, an intense effort resulted in quantifying patient acuity levels and individual staff productivity expectations. This effort was necessary to help quantify staff performance levels, to provide improved measures of productivity, and to systematize before moving into agencywide automation.

THE HI-C'S: BARRIERS TO SUCCESS

Today health care providers are struggling to survive the barriers to success that may be referred to as the hi-c's: costs, competition, and coverage. They are confronted with shrinking human resources and plummeting reimbursement. As demonstrated by the Persian Gulf War, there is an ongoing concern regarding the redirection of vitally needed health care dollars to defense needs and international issues. The federal deficit is not anticipated to become resolved in the near future and everyone will be expected to do more with less financial support from both federal and state governments. Barriers to success include:

1. As health care costs continue to skyrocket, hospitals, as the hub of health care within the community, will seek alternatives for meeting the growing health care needs of their community and to remain competitive within the industry. Deinstitutionalized services such as home care are the only answer in many instances.
2. Competition for staff, for patients, and for health care dollars introduces new challenges for health care providers. Health care, as in political worldwide relationships, offers allies today who may be the greatest competitors tomorrow and vice versa.
3. Coverage issues and concerns relate to both staffing shortages and reimbursement as health care moves even further out of the hands of medical providers into the direct control of payers.

The survival of any hospital-based HHA depends upon the survival of the parent hospital. Therefore, the charge to these HHAs must be to focus attention and resources on determining how to convert any hospital obstacle into an opportunity through home care intervention and support. One of the best examples as to how home care intervention can strengthen any hospital system today is home care involvement as part of the hospital discharge planning process to identify, alleviate, and eliminate any problematic DRG/LOS through expanded home care service programs. The goal of hospital-based home care providers is to ensure that both the hospital and the HHA will survive and flourish now and well into the future.

Since government reimbursement is highly unpredictable, there is a need to develop a variety of alternatives to survive with or without federal funding. For example, without any advanced warning, in July

1985, the federal government changed home care Medicare reimbursement from the aggregate to discipline-specific reimbursement. The impact was devastating to many agencies. Some home care administrators' continued employment was jeopardized as their boards viewed these changes as the result of poor management rather than as an unpredictable and uncontrollable effect. Appropriately positioning the HHA and all the home care product lines within the hospital structure will maximize the financial benefit of the agency to the hospital.

CONTRACTING FOR HOME CARE SERVICES

As home care providers become more involved in hi-tech services, there will be an increasing need to contract new technologies and specialty service staff. All providers should exercise extreme caution when contracting for services and must have profound understanding of changing interpretations of the Internal Revenue Service regulations and applications. It is a catch-22 because government departments do not always agree with each other's requirements. Home care providers must make every effort to comply with each of the government departments' changing mandates and varying perceptions.

Home care providers should focus on and differentiate between an employee and an independent contractor. The IRS has become very stringent in enforcing rulings when there is suspicion that an agency may be using independent contractors to avoid payment of benefits and withholding taxes. The IRS will challenge requirements for independent contractors and for employees, and the employer will need to justify the differences between the two. A key measurement is how much independence contractors have and what are the different expectations and controls imposed upon them. For example, are meetings and inservice requirements the same? Do contractors use agency offices, equipment, and supplies or do they supply their own? Rates could include a separate charge for rental of equipment and use of agency offices, phones, and secretarial staff.

In January 1988, the IRS published 20 criteria and eight specific points necessary to determine independent contractor versus employee status. Some of these criteria are in direct conflict with requirements for agency certification, accreditation, and licensure. The bottom line is control: surveyors are looking for increased control of caregivers, and the IRS is requiring contractors to have less controls imposed upon them. One of the few exceptions that may be considered would be if all HHAs treat independent contractors the same way in any given region. This may be acceptable to the IRS as what is common practice in that particular area. HHAs are encouraged to seek legal advice from a knowledgeable source when assessing compliance and when potential areas of concern are identified.

HOW TO MARKET UNDER MEDICARE

Marketing under the Medicare certified HHA model is far too restrictive. For example, there exists great flexibility for sales and marketing opportunities in the non-Medicare vendor type home care business, affording the private sector a decided edge on the capture of a more sizable share of the home care marketplace. This is of particular significance today with Health Maintenance Organizations (HMOs) and other managed care providers who, in seeking lower-cost providers, are contracting for home care services with less costly, nonregulated staffing vendors, rather than with high-cost, highly regulated, Medicare certified, licensed, and accredited HHAs.

Patient solicitation, sales, and marketing are restricted and a disallowed expense under the Medicare home care program. There is, however, a limited margin of opportunity to engage in some marketing endeavors within an extremely rigid framework. Even though Medicare certified HHAs may not actively solicit patients, and may not engage in extensive advertising, they may provide information and education (and, most of them do this extensively and very effectively).

Home care providers need to know enough to be able to challenge anyone who may want them to implement changes that may have a negative impact on their business. For example, one agency had been confronted by a Medicare state surveyor who insisted that the content of independent contracts should include excerpts from the HHA conditions of participation. The surveyor focused on quality control issues and, therefore, wanted similar requirements for both independent contractors and employees. Since this request could result in costly IRS disallowances, the provider was able to convince the surveyor that the agency had in place sufficient quality control measures with quantifiable expectations and, therefore, did not change existing contracts.

Many hospital systems have widespread ad campaigns that include the HHA along with their other businesses. These types of ad campaigns are an excellent way to convey information about their hospital-based home health agency. There is no industry today as challenging as health care, because providers struggle to provide quality services with limited and rapidly diminishing resources, combined with escalating technological demands. Consumer and referral source education is the effective market tool. Education not only informs the potential customer regarding the HHA's services, but it makes that consumer wiser in the process.

Quality and liability issues must be addressed, and we take an active role in educating HMOs and others as to the differences between various home care provider types. A quote in the October 28, 1988 issue of *Modern Healthcare* stated that, "Most managed care systems emphasize cost cutting at the expense of the patient outcome, thus creating an adversarial relationship with providers." A recent lawsuit filed by NAHC against Health and Human Services on this very issue in only one example reflecting this growing nationwide concern.

There are nonlicensed, non-Medicare certified, nonaccredited staffing agencies accepting chemotherapy, pediatric ventilator patients, and other very sick patients who require extensive home health and high technology services. Referrers and consumers frequently call upon any home care provider that they have heard about through various ads and other marketing endeavors. Some of these agencies do not even provide seven-day per week, 24-hour coverage for these extremely vulnerable patients. Many do not have qualified, experienced back-up staffing support systems. But, these vendor type agencies, in many instances, are able to elicit referrals that should be provided by Medicare-certified HHAs that, in most cases, are better equipped to provide these services. These vendors do extensive sales and marketing of their home care products and services, and many consumers and payors do not know the difference in provider types until it is too late. Many certified and accredited HHAs have received referral of patients after they have been placed in crisis by staffing agencies that were ill-equipped to appropriately care for these very sick patients.

Whether an agency's marketing efforts are overt or covert in nature, knowledge regarding the criteria used by Medicare auditors in evaluating the appropriateness of Medicare-certified HHA's marketing endeavors is essential. They are as follows:

1. Is it solicitation? Is it information and education?
2. What is the reasonableness of monies spent for marketing as it relates to size and scope of agency operation?
3. What is considered to be reasonable marketing practice in your particular area?

Medicare requirements are constantly changing. Even though providers challenge what they feel is inappropriate, they must know all expectations and requirements of the Medicare program and must apprise their staff of any changes on an ongoing basis.

FUTURE DIRECTIONS

Many challenging aspects of home care have been cited in this article, but there are far more positive features to consider. The entire health care industry is moving from an institutional focus to deinstitutionalized services such as ambulatory care, surgi-centers, and free-standing clinics. All of these still take patients away from their homes, and people do prefer all types of home-delivered services, including heath care services.

The future direction of health care is home care. Lifeline links from the home to area emergency rooms are becoming commonplace. Even though home care will never replace the hospital or the nursing home, the key focus of all health care support services and wellness programs of the future will be in the home environment.

The trend for all types of service delivery systems today is in the home. One can pay bills and order needed items and services without leaving home. TV home shopping is already a big business; Pizza Hut, a leader in the pizza market, soon discovered that their future survival depended upon home-delivered pizzas. If parents live away from their children, the children can arrange for a variety of services including home maintenance, snow removal, pet-sitting and plant care services, and bath and tuck-in services to help maintain their parents at home.

As hospital technology becomes even more sophisticated, there will be a corollary expansion of these services in home care and these services will become even more accessible. As astronauts are monitored in space, this technology can also be applied to monitor cardiac patients in their homes with holter monitors or telephone telemetry. Biotelemetry services of all types will soon be commonplace in home care. Telecommunication devices, such as those used for the deaf, transport electronic signals over telephone wires. Diagnostic and treatment technology will be expanded through advanced telemetry. Robotics is evolving as another form of high technology to monitor vital signs and dispense medications in the home. The number of new and expanded Medicare and non-Medicare home care businesses will continue to skyrocket. Home care-oriented businesses will be on every corner in communities of the future.

19

Competition in Accrediting: Letting Other Voices Be Heard

Clark C. Havighurst

*P*erhaps the lowest common denominator of the membership of the National League for Nursing (NLN) is resistance to the medical profession's paradigm of health care. Under this paradigm physicians make all important decisions, individually or collectively, with as few financial constraints and as little input from consumers and other interests as possible. If the raison d'être of the NLN does indeed include opposition to some values and views held by physicians, then the NLN may have some very valuable opinions to express on subjects cutting across the entire spectrum of health care issues. Accreditation of educational and service delivery programs provides an ideal opportunity for an organization like the NLN to express its uniquely informed views about such things as what constitutes quality in health care, what is truly valuable to patients, and the vital trade-offs that must be faced if consumers and taxpayers are to get good value for the vast amounts they spend on health services.

A few years ago, the NLN created the Community Health Accreditation Program (CHAP) to accredit home health agencies and home care providers. The decision to make CHAP a largely independent entity, with strong representation of consumers and purchasers on its board, reveals the intention of the NLN to create a counterweight to other accrediting programs and regulatory regimes. Because other accrediting and regulatory programs exist under different sponsorship, they may neglect certain values such as emphasizing the discrete inputs of home care while disregarding the quality of life of home care patients. Even if the intention of the NLN's program is to supply what some might call a gold standard, reflecting the highest

147

aspirations of the nursing profession and some consumer interests rather than merely minimum standards of acceptable home care, the NLN's contribution can still be very valuable. We need such benchmarks of excellence even if economic and other constraints prevent the NLN's ideals from being realized everywhere or in every financing program. I sense that CHAP sees itself as the conscience of the home health care industry and is filling this role with distinction.

The NLN has apparently not defined its goal as monopolizing accreditation in the home health field. On the contrary, it recognizes that some competition is inevitable and it wants only a chance to offer its accrediting services in a fair competitive environment. At the moment, the NLN faces very intense competition from another accreditor, the Joint Commission on Accreditation of Healthcare Organizations. The Joint Commission is accustomed to monopolizing the accreditation of hospitals and does not shrink from aspiring to a dominant role in other fields as well. At the end of this chapter, I will address the ongoing contest between CHAP and the Joint Commission from the point of view of antitrust law. First, however, I want to discuss competition and monopoly in accrediting and comparable activities in more general terms. My purpose is to identify the policy arguments for competition in these activities and some potential issues under antitrust law. One reason why I make reference only to potential legal issues is that, although I may see some serious antitrust problems here, many other analysts would not acknowledge any antitrust problem at all. Indeed, much of what I say here is only a minority view of the law, not so much because my views have been analyzed and rejected but rather because no one has really put them to the test. In any event, the more important thing may not be the legal question as such but the case I want to make for competition in private accrediting, private credentialing, and private certification—indeed in private standard-setting and seal of approval activities of all kinds.

THE JOINT COMMISSION AS A LEGALLY QUESTIONABLE JOINT VENTURE

Let me begin by identifying a problem—I see it as an antitrust problem—concerning the Joint Commission's status as the dominant accreditor of hospitals in the United States. The Joint Commission is a joint venture of several powerful sponsoring organizations, specifically, the American Medical Association, the American Hospital Association, the American College of Physicians, and the American College of Surgeons. An antitrust lawyer confronting such a joint venture should automatically ask whether the coming together of independent entities in a common enterprise is compatible with the maintenance of vigorous competition in the affected market. The policy declared in the Sherman Act is that competition in decentralized markets is society's chosen instrument for advancing consumer welfare. Furthermore, claims that competition should be restricted in order to achieve some generally worthy purpose or some greater good must be addressed to legislatures instead of the courts. The Joint Commission should therefore be scrutinized solely to determine its effects on competition as a process that effectively diffuses and checks the exercise of private power.

Most antitrust experts viewing the Joint Commission would say that competition is generally helped, not hurt, by the valuable advice concerning hospital quality that it provides to the marketplace. Still, I would go farther than most of these experts and argue that a valid joint venture to produce such advice should not have to justify in court (except in general terms) the standards it uses in making its judgments. Even though providers who are adversely affected will often wish to bring antitrust suits questioning the basis for, and the motives behind, the opinions that a joint venture expresses, the mere publication of an opinion cannot, in itself, harm the competitive process by retraining trade. When the Joint Commission was sued a few years back for maintaining an accrediting standard implying that a good hospital would never allow nonphysicians (clinical psychologists and podiatrists, for example) to belong to its medical staff, I would have defended the Joint Commission's right to hold and base accrediting decisions on that opinion. I would have disagreed with that view and argued that it reflected the Joint Commission's domination by physicians; nevertheless, I would have defended a joint venture's legal right to say what most of its members probably believed. Moreover, I would not have had to rely on the constitutional freedom of speech in reaching this legal conclusion. Within very wide limits, self-interested collective speech and open criticism of competitors are entirely compatible with vigorous competition.

My legal objections to the Joint Commission thus have nothing to do with the positions it takes on particular issues. Instead, I am concerned about the monopoly of opinion that results when several entities, holding and capable of expressing different or competing views on what makes a good hospital, combine to speak with one voice. In a 1983 article, Nancy King and I argued that the Joint Commission constitutes a combination in restraint of trade because it comprises the four health care organizations in the best position to form and express authoritative, independent opinions about hospital quality. We took the position that such joint venture should be condemned under the Sherman Act precisely because it precludes and suppresses competition in the production of commercially valuable information and opinion. We did not mean to imply that, in the absence of the Joint Commission, each of its four constituent bodies would maintain a hospital accrediting program of its own; that would be most unlikely because of the economies of scale in accrediting. But, one of the four, for example, the American Medical Association, would probably take over the Joint Commission's operating. It would not be implausible to expect one of the remaining organizations, for example, the American Hospital Association, to organize an alternative accrediting program if its members found the surviving program to be objectionable in some major respect.

In any event, competition of the kind I value could exist even if only one of the four former sponsors of the Joint Commission maintained an independent program of hospital accreditation. That program would have to recognize the possibility that a competing program might be started if there were too much dissatisfaction with its performance. (Antitrust lawyers recognize the bracing effect of such potential competition in other concentrated markets.) In addition, such an accreditor could not hope to enjoy the same prestige and dominance as the Joint Commission, if only because the other three would be constantly sniping at it, publicly criticizing its policies, and alerting the public to its possible biases and to the existence of different, strongly held opinions on vital matters. There would, in other words, be more competition, more information and more open debate about hospitals, than there is today. I strongly believe that antitrust law should be invoked to preserve and protect competition in the production of information and opinion, to foster competition in what is in many crucial respects a marketplace of ideas about what constitutes good medical care. Antitrust enforcers and courts should remember that control of information is a key to power and that the antitrust laws were enacted to prevent the accumulation of undue, unchecked power in the private economy.

Before I leave this subject, let me suggest some consequences of the Joint Commission's monopoly of hospital accreditation. A majority of the sponsors of the Joint Commission are physician organizations; a majority of its individual members are physicians representing the interests and views of the practicing profession. It is therefore no coincidence that the Joint Commission's standards for hospital accreditation are so heavily focused on ensuring the dominance of physicians in hospitals. Instead of attempting to evaluate hospitals on the basis of patient outcomes (only recently the Joint Commission has begun to inquire into patient experiences in hospitals), the Joint Commission long concentrated exclusively on structural matters, particularly on ensuring a major role in hospital governance for self-governing medical staffs. The Joint Commission has thus used its strategic position to foster the medical profession's paradigmatic view that all decisions affecting medical care in hospitals should be made by, or in coequal collaboration with, an independently organized, unaccountable medical staff.

It is not an a priori necessity that physicians should enjoy in every hospital the extraordinary privilege of self-governance. Indeed, in few enterprises does one find administrative subdivisions electing their own officers or a similar, pervasive private requirement that the enterprise be operated as a joint venture of independent entities rather than as a single integrated firm. The universal practice of allowing physicians to enjoy self-governance and to exercise the resulting power in hospitals is largely an artifact of physician dominance of the Joint Commission and of the Joint Commission's ability to dictate the limits of innovation in structuring the relationship between hospital and physician. I truly regret that antitrust law has never been employed to contest this monopoly over the definition of standards for American hospitals.

THE IMPLICATIONS OF APPLYING ANTITRUST LAW TO COLLABORATION IN ACCREDITING

It should now be easy to see why there has not been much official support for my view that potential competitors collaborating in the operation of an accrediting program should be subject to scrutiny under the antitrust laws. The implications of adopting my analysis are so subversive of the medical profession's power, and would necessitate such a radical departure from the accepted paradigm of medical decision making, that few have been willing to take the leap and consider my antitrust agenda. Indeed, if antitrust enforcers accepted my view that the private production of commercially significant information and opinion constitutes trade or commerce subject to policing under the Sherman Act, there would be a long list of candidates for legal challenge, each of them a sacred cow of the highest order. Government officials who undertook to challenge any one of them would have to face public criticism and significant political risks. Although the Justice Department's recent attack on the Ivy League as a price-fixing cartel may suggest a new courageousness among antitrust enforcers, those officials would still be fearful of trying to explain their rationale for attacking conspiracies that affect only the output of information and opinion, not price.

Accrediting and credentialing monopolies resulting from joint ventures similar to the Joint Commission exist throughout the health care sector, depriving the public at almost every point of the opportunity to hear and act upon unapproved, alternative views on a myriad of cumulatively important questions. Let me run quickly through my list of candidates for antitrust scrutiny as way of demonstrating how antitrust enforcement of competition in accrediting could introduce a desirable dose of pluralism in the health care sector. Even if antitrust law cannot be relied upon to restore pluralism, *glasnost* can be introduced into the health care system in other ways, permitting for the first time some effective challenges to the medical profession's one-party rule and control of information. Too many crucial issues are being resolved in back rooms by elite groups like the Joint Commission and not in the free marketplace. This is not, I submit, the American way.

Many of the instrumentalities by which organized medicine gives effect to its views on crucial matters relate to the credentialing of personnel to work in the health care industry. Medical specialists are certified through programs operated under the umbrellas of the American Board of Medical Specialties and the Council of Medical Specialty Societies. These collaborative bodies closely coordinate the actions of their constituent organizations, ensuring that none of them embarks on an independent path such as encroaching on the turf of a sister specialty. Similar arrangements exist in dentistry. In the allied health occupations, the overall situation is more difficult to assess, but the medical profession has its hands in many credentialing pies. Although many issues encountered in these areas are of limited overall consequence, organized medicine maintains its presence in these fields in order to block actions that might threaten physician interests such as expanding an occupation's scope of independent practice.

Personnel credentialing is always closely linked with educational matters and the medical profession dominates educational accrediting in most health care fields. The Liaison Committee on Medical Education, which accredits medical schools, is a joint venture of the American Medical Association and the Association of American Medical Colleges. Under the Liaison Committee on Medical Education's hegemony, there have long been significant ideological limits on how tomorrow's doctors could be trained. As an illustration of this point consider whether the Kaiser-Permanente Medical School, dedicated to preparing students for cost-conscious prepaid group practices, would have had an easy time getting accredited in the last 40 years. In the legal profession, the American Bar Association and the Association of American Law Schools maintain separate accrediting programs. Not only does this demonstrate that concurrent accrediting efforts can coexist in professional fields, but there is more diversity in legal education than there has ever been in medical training since educational accrediting began.

Graduate training for physicians is accredited almost exclusively by cooperating medical organizations closely linked to the medical profession's mechanisms for certifying specialists. The field of continuing medical education, although it receives little public attention, has seen a series of joint ventures and mergers over the years, with periodic outbreaks of competition. Education in many allied health occupations is presided over by accreditors sponsored jointly by the American Medical Association and the dominant occupational group in the particular field. An exception to the medical profession's usual dominance, which convincingly demonstrates the significance of its general influence, appears in the field of physical therapy, where some years ago the American Medical Association and American Physical Therapy Association had a falling out. That schism resulted to some extent in training for therapists that prepares, and thus induces, them to aspire to wider roles, including independent practice.

Once the full extent of the medical profession's standard-setting and informational role is understood, is it any wonder that physicians' paradigm of medical care is so well entrenched in the health care industry as a whole? Although accrediting and credentialing seemingly involve nothing more than the expression of authoritative opinions concerning appropriate conduct by industry participants, the domination of these activities by the private medical profession gives it the quasi-regulatory power it needs to avert or channel much unwanted change. I see no good policy or legal reason why the antitrust laws should not be used to contest monopolistic control of these crucial informational activities. But even if antitrust intervention is not in the cards, there are many other opportunities for government to encourage competing organizations to enter the market and offer alternative accrediting and credentialing services. Let me now turn to a policy discussion of the merits of competition in accrediting and government's current attitude with regard to such competition.

ACCREDITATION IN POLICY PERCEPTIVE

The arguments against competition in accrediting frequently include the observation that economies of scale and the economics of public goods may dictate that only one effective, high quality accreditor can exist or is needed in any discrete field. That argument assumes, however, that each accreditor is doing exactly the same thing: applying agreed-upon standards to the same set of providers. But different accreditors may employ different standards, thus performing different rather than duplicative services for the consuming public. Although economics will certainly limit the number of competitors, there is room for competition as long as there is a demand for alternative points of view on relevant issues. There is also, to be sure, the usual public good problem: the weakening of incentives for private production of valuable information that results from the difficulty of excluding free riders from using such information without paying for it. But even though information, as a public good, will always be chronically underproduced in a free market (unless public subsidies are provided), there will always be some demand for accrediting by candidates for accreditation, which may value it as an aid in marketing themselves to wary consumers and other purchasers, including government. That this is a market in which output and competition will always be suboptimal is no reason why we should not seek as much output and competition as we can get.

Another common argument against competition in accrediting is that consumers will be confused and will not know which accreditors to trust. Ironically, accreditors face the same problem that is faced by those whom they accredit: the consumer does not know whom to trust. Thus, there is a need for some accreditation of the accreditors themselves. In the field of education, the Department of Education provides such an accrediting service by itself formally recognizing private accreditors of educational programs. (The NLN enjoys such recognition in the field of nursing education.) Although primarily designed to ensure that federal funds are given only to reputable educational programs, the Department's oversight of educational accreditors also gives the general public some assurance that a particular accreditation means something more than possession of a fancy seal.

Unfortunately, the Department of Education has not always fostered competition among educational accrediting bodies but has tended instead to enfranchise a single accreditor for each type of educational program in each geographic area. In 1988, however, the Department, in adopting new regulations, rejected suggestions that it should avoid public confusion by expressly discouraging competition among accreditors. The following statement by the Department, in publishing its final regulations, is significant:

> With regard to the use of the regulations to limit proliferation and fragmentation in accreditation, the Secretary [then William Bennett] determined that arbitrarily limiting the number of accrediting bodies serves no educational purpose. The Secretary wishes to foster appropriate competition among accrediting bodies and does not wish to see the recognition process used in such a way as to create a monopoly in any educational field.

The Health Care Financing Administration (HCFA) gives private accreditors a comparable role in evaluating the eligibility of health care providers to participate in federal programs. A hospital's accreditation by the Joint Commission has long been deemed to establish its compliance with Medicare's conditions of participation, subject to occasional verification by government and spot checks in response to complaints. In 1987, HCFA proposed—it has not yet taken final action—to give similar recognition to the NLN's accreditation of home health agencies. Under proposed regulations issued last December, HCFA would invite private accrediting organizations to apply for the power to grant deemed status to a wide variety of other providers. Neither Congress nor HCFA has ever expressly said, however, that competition in accrediting is to be encouraged. Nevertheless, the American Osteopathic Association has long been recognized as a second accreditor of hospitals. Clinical laboratories are subject to accreditation by a number of private organizations as a substitute for federal licensure. And, HCFA has expressly contemplated that both the Joint Commission and CHAP might accredit home health agencies for Medicare. HCFA's primary purpose, like that of the Department of Education, is to ensure that the federal government does business only with reputable service providers. But, the general public would also benefit from the agency's verification of the reliability of particular accreditation programs.

There is one difference between the uses of private accreditation by the Department of Education and HCFA that suggests some limits on the potential role of competition in accrediting in the health care field. Partly because the First Amendment precludes direct federal control of education, the Department of Education has not sought to impose its own regulatory standards on educational programs, but has chosen instead to accept the judgments of reputable accrediting programs, which use standards of their own making. HCFA, on the other hand, looks to private accreditors to determine whether federal standards (e.g., Medicare's conditions of participation) have been met. One might therefore view HCFA's enlistment of private accreditors as a kind of privatization of the enforcement of public standards. The Department of Education, on the other hand, has delegated the standard-setting function itself.

In practice, however, this difference may not be as great as first appears. In its 1987 proposal to recognize both the NLN's and the Joint Commission's accrediting programs for home health care, HCFA seemed willing to overlook major differences between Medicare's written standards and the requirements of the respective private accreditors. In so doing, it stressed that the important thing was not the precise requirements enforced or the precise procedures followed but the general reliability of the private organization to detect deficient services. HCFA's ability to verify and look behind the private accreditor's decisions and to investigate particular complaints was deemed to provide an ample opportunity for the government to enforce its own particular requirements. The striking thing is that HCFA seemed willing to trust the private organization's application of its own standards in the first instance. I do understand, of course, that the Reagan administration was probably more permissive in this respect than other administrations are likely to be. Moreover, since 1987 CHAP has tailored many of its accreditation requirements and procedures to resemble HCFA's requirements and procedures more closely than they did originally. It is quite possible that such competition as may emerge in the accrediting of home heath agencies may yet turn out, because of federal insistence that the job be done exactly its way, to preclude significant diversity in judging quality.

The Reagan administration's proposal in the early 1980s to accept Joint Commission accreditation of nursing homes sheds some additional light on the distinction between privatization of the enforcement function and delegation of broader responsibilities. That proposal was widely criticized in Congress and elsewhere by persons who viewed it as an abdication of government's responsibility for the quality of care in nursing homes. The concept of reliance on private accreditors has not been revived with respect to nursing homes even though it was endorsed with respect to numerous other providers in HCFA's proposal of December, 1991. Because of the great public sensitivity about nursing home quality, private accreditation is not likely soon to substitute for direct public control in this field. Nevertheless, private accreditation of nursing homes should still be pursued because it supplements public regulation and can contribute to pluralism, especially if competing accreditors emerge.

In my view, there should nearly always be room in health care fields, as there is in education, for government to rely on private accreditors, applying their own standards, to determine eligibility to participate in public programs. Instead of prescribing detailed, explicit standards itself, government could usually discharge its responsibility for ensuring a minimum standard of quality by recognizing competing accreditors, not as later egos enforcing the government's will but as trustworthy watchdogs for consumer interests. Direct regulation is often heavy-handed and less efficacious in achieving desired levels of meaningful quality than private accrediting might be. In addition, the different standards that different accreditors may apply may reflect different subjective preferences that exist within the population. Within limits, public programs should be willing to accommodate such preferences. Allowing competing, reputable private accreditors to verity the acceptability of particular providers as options for consumers is an effective way of preserving pluralism that is otherwise hard to maintain in public programs. Moreover, such private accreditors, themselves accredited by government, can simultaneously serve the private sector as sources of reliable information and opinion on matters of technical complexity and great importance to consumers. I am pleased to see the NLN taking the lead in demonstrating that alternative accreditors can provide the assurances that government needs to run its programs without becoming simply another arm of heavy-handed government.

THE NLN VERSUS THE JOINT COMMISSION

Let me now turn to the problems that CHAP is currently encountering in its efforts to compete with the Joint Commission in accrediting home health agencies. The Joint Commission has determined that, if a hospital it is accrediting has a well defined ongoing relationship with a home health care provider or agency, its surveyors must satisfy themselves concerning that agency or provider before it can accredit the hospital. The Joint Commission's position is that it accredits total programs and that, if the hospital in any way represents that its services include home health care, its arrangements for providing that care must be reviewed. Although the Joint Commission's position is logical at first glance, it raises some serious problems for both home health agencies and the NLN—and very likely, it also raises serious problems for the Joint Commission itself under antitrust law.

The Joint Commission's policy creates a powerful inducement for a home health agency to seek accreditation by the Joint Commission rather than by CHAP. Once a home health agency is accredited by the Joint Commission, it does not have to be surveyed anew every time a hospital with which it has an arrangement comes up for survey. Accreditation by the Joint Commission also makes an agency especially attractive to hospitals as a joint venture partner. Not only does it enjoy the Joint Commission's seal of approval, but it can offer the hospital relief from the Joint Commission's charge for the extra survey. A number of visiting nurse associations and other home health providers are feeling pressure from hospitals to seek accreditation by the Joint Commission. Few of them would be likely to pay for accreditation by CHAP as well.

Without trying to sort out all the legalities, let me observe that the Joint Commission appears to have created what antitrust lawyers call a tying arrangement. In effect, it is saying to hospitals, "If you want our accreditation for your hospital, you must either pay us to survey any suppliers with which you have subcontracts or persuade them to buy our separate accreditation service." Tying arrangements are generally unlawful if the seller possesses substantial market power in the market for the tying product—in this case, hospital accreditation—and uses it to force another product—the tied product—on the consumer. Because the Joint Commission so obviously dominates the market for hospital accreditation, a court might well see its requirements with respect to home health care as an exercise of unlawful leverage. The Joint Commission's defense of its policy would probably fail to convince an antitrust court, despite its apparent logic, because it neglects the obvious alternative of recognizing accreditation by CHAP as a partial or complete substitute for a Joint Commission survey.

Unfortunately, litigating such manners is never easy or cheap. There would be a number of complex questions that would have to be resolved before the Joint Commission could be forced through litigation to mend its ways. Nevertheless, I think a lawsuit against the Joint Commission could be successful. It would be easier to find a violation here than in a recent case in Florida, *Key Enterprises, Inc. v. Venice Hospital.* In that case, a monopoly hospital was found to have unlawfully used its leverage to steer patients in need of home care following their hospitalization to an affiliated supplier of durable medical equipment. The crucial difficulty was that home health nurses felt some pressure to recommend the hospital's preferred supplier over its competitor, even though the hospital had refrained from exerting its leverage overtly. The Joint Commission's use of leverage is not nearly so subtle, and the monopoly power it wields is legally more questionable (for reasons indicated above) than that possessed by Venice Hospital.

I have some serious reservations about the result in the *Key Enterprises, Inc. v. Venice Hospital* case as well as about many other decisions condemning tying arrangements and other techniques by which a monopoly in one field is allegedly parlayed into another monopoly or into an unfair competitive advantage in another market. Nevertheless, because the Joint Commission's dubious monopoly over the supply of information about hospitals is apparently unassailable by any other legal means, I am able to overcome my usual doctrinal scruples about such cases and would encourage any efforts CHAP might make to obtain fairer treatment at the hands of its competitor. In any legal attack that might be mounted on CHAP's behalf, however, the complaint should not concede (as most antitrust lawyers would be inclined to do) the lawfulness of the Joint Commission's monopoly over the tying product, the accreditation of hospitals. Although the illegality of that monopoly is not an essential predicate for your cause of action under current doctrine, it should be prominently and forcefully alleged in order to strengthen your case, to encourage the Joint Commission to accept an early settlement, and to identify for the larger public an issue of immense importance in American health care.

I will watch this area with interest for further developments, just as I will watch the NLN's continuing efforts to establish the value and legitimacy of competition in accrediting in home health care and other fields. The NLN's independent voice should continue to be heard throughout the health care sector.

PART EIGHT

Reevaluating Nursing's Agenda

20

Presidential Address for the Biennial Convention

Patty Hawken

*I*t seems like yesterday that I was standing here before you ready to assume the presidency of this organization. I am here at the end of this presidency to report to you on our activities during this past biennium and to enumerate what we have accomplished.

Let me begin by saying I have enjoyed serving as your president and representing you at a myriad of activities—from lunch with Barbara Bush to celebrate National Nurses' Week in 1990 to serving on the Tri-Council to attending state league conventions. The two years as president have been busy and exhilarating for me.

Never before has there been such an exciting time for the nursing community. Never before have we had such a golden opportunity to rise to the fore and achieve a very influential position in health care delivery. The opportunity presented itself in the form of a health care delivery system floundering in disarray. The lack of leadership in health care delivery made it patently clear that nurses could move in and fill the gap and provide the leadership so badly needed.

I am extremely pleased that during this biennium, the National League for Nursing has demonstrated that leadership and advanced a national health proposal for the nursing community to consider and ultimately to support. I am referring to our Nursing Agenda for Health Care Reform. NLN initiated the proposal to bring to the nursing community and, joined by the American Nurse Association, has now developed nursing's proposal. As of this date, over 40 organizations have endorsed it. This means close to one million nurses are standing together on a single nursing initiative. It has to be a first, and an exciting first for nurses to join together in a proactive way. In the

161

past, we joined together in a reactive way to thwart the Registered Care Technologist (RCT) proposal and to remove *Nightingales* from TV. As you read the Nursing Agenda, there will be questions: how will it begin, how much will it cost, and so forth. We have some answers, but purposefully did not put everything into this proposal, since it is a political document and as such it needs to be broad based and open to political input.

We must now take our message to the public and then to Congress. In order for nursing's agenda to be meaningful, we must have strategies in place, in schools and in constituent leagues across the nation, to educate and strike chords of response in the public and professional arena.

The uniqueness of nursing's position must be our commitment to change and our ability to build a constituency for our reform agenda. We must wage a campaign that advances a new health care delivery system that is *affordable, accessible,* and of *high quality.* We need to share our thoughts with each other, other professionals and, of course, consumers. We need to present and commit ourselves to a new paradigm shift.

Clearly, we need an entirely new view of the world, a new framework for looking at things, and nursing's agenda can provide that framework: That is the mission of our agenda for health care reform; and quality health care education and service are the main missions of the National League for Nursing.

I have a vision: Nursing Agenda for Health Care Reform becomes a bill in Congress. All constituent leagues and members work with legislators, consumers, neighbors and the bill is passed. I envision nursing leaders gathered around the President as he flourishes 20 pens to sign the bill and hands them out. I envision over two million nurses feeling proud and excited that they made a difference and will continue to make a difference on the health of this nation. You may say, "What did you put in your orange juice this morning?" If we set high standards and goals, we can achieve high standards and goals. If we settle for lower goals, we will always function in mediocrity. NLN will set its standards high!

Through several key programs and key initiatives, we have been working to improve the quality of health care by shifting the paradigm:

- First, we are working to position our network of community nursing centers as key components of the delivery system: (1) by improving basic access to health care for all populations, (2) by establishing community nursing centers throughout this nation, and (3) by staffing these centers with prepared nurse practitioners. This would change the entire focus and framework of health care: a paradigm shift.
- Second, we are working to establish our community health accreditation program as the accrediting body of choice in the out-of-hospital arena, where nurses will have a prominent voice in

the quality of care delivered. By establishing standards and maintaining these standards, nurses have a direct impact on home health and nursing home care. And so far, this effort has been successful: another paradigm shift.

- Third, we are working to position nurses as mainstream providers of care—as case managers, as clinical specialists, the new gateopeners not gatekeepers of the system—coordinating care and determining its reasonable cost and appropriateness. We believe that nurses can and do provide cost-effective, quality care and it is time we demonstrated that ability nationwide: third paradigm shift.

- And finally, we are working to design a socially, fiscally, and academically sound system of nursing education that is publicly accountable for our graduates, who are prepared not only to deliver knowledgeable, compassionate, and skillful care in today's system but to also assume the necessary leadership for the future of health care in this country.

These are four key initiatives, aimed at fundamental reform that will effect the paradigm shift we need so badly in the health care delivery; a shift in which community-based models of care, nurses as primary care givers, and nursing curricula focused on prevention and community care will prevail.

Because the League is known best for its educational mission, it is important to remember that it is in the educational arena where we have the greatest opportunity of all to hasten the movement to a new paradigm.

In order to prepare practitioners in nursing suited to assume these new roles, nursing education must become more relevant and responsive to society's needs for reform. As the Carnegie Report compellingly phrased it, "problems in health care cry out for faculty solutions" and I will hasten to add, nursing faculty specifically.

College and university settings have always been centers for social change, for innovation, centers of discovery. Now we are badly in need of new ways of doing things, new ways of solving our health care dilemma. It is time to bring our campaign for reform to the campus, to create the momentum to achieve an effective system of health care delivery. The momentum to shift the paradigm can be created in three key ways:

- *First, through nursing education programs that are increasingly socially relevant:* We need vital new curricula that come alive with the understanding and knowledge of health care problems in our communities. We need new relationships between nursing faculty and consumer groups committed to the changes needed in health care. We must form partnerships with our community colleagues and our nursing service counterparts and seek and incorporate their ideas and needs in our curricula.

- *Second, through new clinical experiences:* The hospital of today represents one method of health care delivery, usually acute care. Hospitals are not readily equipped to care for chronic disease, rehabilitation, or to prevent disease in the first place. We want to maintain hospital experiences for students, however, our students' clinical experiences should reflect new directions and be predominantly in home care, long-term care settings, in nursing clinics, and in community health centers. Health care delivery is moving away from the costly inpatient setting and our clinical experiences should reflect these trends.

- *Third, through our students:* We graduate about 60,000 new students a year, new professionals who enter the delivery system. We have an opportunity to teach them to apply pressure in the system where it will do the most good. We have the opportunity, as this membership affirmed in passing the resolution in 1989 entitled "Innovative Curricula," to teach our students how to transform the health care system into one more reflective of nursing's values. We can teach students to focus on the economics of health care on behalf of patients. We can teach them to focus on quality in terms of appropriateness and outcomes. And, we can teach them to focus on effecting key legislative changes such as establishing third party payment for nurses or public disclosure laws that would make health care information available to the public. Perhaps most importantly, we can teach them the infinite benefits to all of acknowledging and embracing the full diversity of our society.

We have, in this biennium, accomplished our primary aim: shaping a major agenda for health care reform, nursing's agenda. It is a blueprint to use in your teaching, in your practice, in your communities. This agenda will hopefully serve as the League's roadmap in shaping its programs and priorities in years to come. This agenda will hopefully by one that the American people will come to know and embrace in the not-too-distant future.

As your president, there have been other major aims I have had during this biennium. The first I shall mention is to develop rational guidelines for how to most effectively utilize the graduates we prepare. I am referring to the educational competencies that the League is well known for. It has been striking that during this critical period of the nursing shortage—when nurse executives and policy makers have sought guidance as to the most efficient models of utilization and the best models of differentiated practice—our competencies had little to add to the discussion. As the leader in nursing education, I believe strongly that it is the NLN that should provide the guidance that the nation needs for the efficient and effective utilization of scarce nursing resources.

To that end, during this biennium, we established a task force, broadly representative, to develop a new clear set of competencies that differentiate the abilities of our graduates and provide the guidance that is needed. The final report should come to you sometime before the end of this year. Preliminary results indicate that it will provide the necessary leadership to give guidance in the more efficient utilization of nurses in the future. The initial effort is to differentiate four levels of competency: licensed vocational nurse, diploma or associate degree nurse, bachelor of science nurse, and master of science nurse.

The second aim was to inaugurate the new structure of the NLN and we have done this with a functioning Board of Trustees of the National League Health Council, Inc. and a very active and productive Board of Governors of the NLN. The new structure appears to serve the organization very well and I am pleased to report that all the committees and councils have been very active and productive as you will learn from their reports.

My third and major aim, and most important of all, has been to improve the communication with all of you, the members. It has been my strongly held conviction that the League is only as strong as its members and we have strong members. But, the messages and information about major initiatives and programs to members had not been loud enough or frequent enough to ensure full membership involvement and participation.

Many of you have commented that you see a change and we have worked hard to make that change. We instituted a monthly president's column in *Nursing & Health Care* and we now are on a schedule to bring a key communication to you on a monthly basis. We sent out frequent policy statements, executive wires, NLN updates. I was able to attend several state league conventions, as have staff, and enjoyed meeting and interacting with members. Communication is the lifeblood of every membership organization. I hope that you will continue to see improvement in this critical area in the future.

Many other initiatives were accomplished. We met our accrediting bodies directive by establishing new accreditation outcomes. The accreditation committee is looking at realigning criteria so we see an orderly progression and some commonality between educational councils, review of constitution and bylaws. Education funding and legislative initiatives were pushed forward and many more activities undertaken.

Now as the League grows in stature, in its financial base and in its influence, a strong membership base will be vital to this success. To that end, we are initiating another membership campaign to attract nurses to our mission of quality education and health care delivery. I will never grow tired of saying that I think the National League for Nursing and nursing in this country are on the crest of great things. I believe this biennium—our initiation into the decade of the 90s—has launched us into an exciting agenda for nursing: leading the nation in health care reform.

It has been most exciting for me to serve you in working to shape that agenda and I look forward to continuing that work with all of you, as a proud member of our wonderful profession, and of this great organization.

21

Community-Based Nursing Education in El Salvador

Rosa Rodriguez-Deras

The school of Medical Technology at the University of El Salvador, one of two schools in the Faculty of Medicine, offers nine tracks in health. Nursing, diet and nutrition, health education, ecotechnology and clinical laboratory are offered at the bachelor's degree level. Maternal-child health, physical therapy, radiotechnology, and anesthesiology are offered at the diploma degree level.

The School of Medical Technology was founded in 1973 on the ecological paradigm of Leavell and Clark. In 1983, in an effort to reaffirm its relevance, the school rethought its curriculum with a special focus that would respond to the health needs of the majority of the country's population as expressed in its epidemiological profile.

As stated, the goal of the School of Medical Technology is to implement an integration of the basic functions of research, teaching, and social service. It has opted for making the wellness–illness continuum the general object of study and for carrying out the educational process in its place of origin.

Over the past five years, curriculum tracks relevant to the above statement of goal orientation have evolved in practice. This experience has enriched the interrelationship of students, faculty, and administrators. In designing curriculum together, they have succeeded in making it more functional by evaluating it in the process of their own participation.

By sharing our experiences within the context of the Faculty of Medicine as a whole, we also enrich ourselves with the perspectives of other health disciplines. By sharing our difficulties, which have limited the extent and speed of curriculum development, we enhance our particular perspective.

THEORETICAL FRAMEWORK AND POINT OF REFERENCE

The National Reality and Health Needs

According to historians, at the time of the Spanish conquest of the Americas, a self-sustaining agricultural structure had existed for many centuries. Although the Pipil Indian society was structured into classes—nobles, plebians, merchants, and slaves—work was organized communally and property was held in common. The extreme brutality and rapidity of the Spanish conquest, however, had two immediate effects: it transformed the indigenous population as a whole into a subsurvient class and it resulted in the mixing of races.

After the conquest, in a belated effort to re-establish communal lands for the indigenous population, Crown properties, the "encomienda," were founded. In 1520, this system was converted into "haciendas," properties owned by Spanish settlers. Under the hacienda system feudal relations of production were maintained: the indigenous population was granted communal use of land only in exchange for free or cheap manual labor upon it.

From 1720–1821, the agro-export "latifundia" model came into being and was consolidated via the profitable production of sugar cane, coca, cotton, and indigo. Indigo, a major cash crop, was sold to the European market until the discovery of synthetic dyes. With the resulting loss of the indigo market came the cultivation of coffee, which initiated an indigenous capital model with its dominant oligarchic structure and its dehumanizing ideological orientation toward the exterior.

In 1895, institutionalized health care began in El Salvador with the sanitation of shipping ports as a measure to protect the quality and flow of import-export goods. In 1924, health care became the responsibility of the General Board of Health under the secretary of health. In 1948, due to the development of the important cities of San Salvador, Santa Ana, and San Miguel, health care finally came into its own with the establishment of the Ministry of Public Health and Social Welfare.

During the 1950s and 1960s, a burgeoning international coffee market allowed surplus capital to be reoriented toward industry. As a result, a free trade zone with incentives for foreign capital came into being. To support this trend, the Salvadorian Institute of Social Service (ISSS) was created with the goal of rapid reintegration of urban labor. However, as coffee continued as *the* monocrop at the mercy of the international market, worldwide economic crises wrecked havoc with the country's socioeconomic system.

Due to a lack of development in rural areas where 60 percent of the population lived, the general subsistence economy weakened. For large families, in fact, production decreased below subsistence levels. Migration from the countryside to the cities began en masse. This phenomenon resulted in a peasant workforce without technical skills and little understanding of wage structures living in various "belts of misery" around the cities and unable to meet even their basic needs. The resultant marginal population still suffers chronic hunger; first, second, and third degree infant malnutrition; high maternal and child mortality; and low birth-weight children resulting in impaired physical and mental development. The epidemiological profile has always been led by communicable diseases, underscored by some level of malnutrition and stress which are products of the low standard of living and, of course, the civil war.

In this context, Salvadorian society had exhausted its ability to maintain social equilibrium. In 1979, then, there rose a demand to modify social structures. Although measures were made to appease the population, these were cosmetic in nature but with a revolutionary patina—for example, the Agrarian Reform, which was also part of the counterinsurgency project. However, these changes did little to stop the popular movement nor did they alter the fundamentally unjust and exploitive relationships in society, the true cause of the current conflict which, while ongoing for more than a decade, has further lowered the general standard of living.*

The epidemiological profile has continued to show gastrointestinal illness and acute respitory infections as leading cases of morbidity; certain effects of the prenatal period have also raised indices of infant mortality. Parallel to this health situation, the services offered by the Ministry of Health are limited. Further attacks against the economic system also lower the number of people served by the Salvadorian Institute of Social Security. Access to private service, on the other hand, is available only to the small number of users capable of paying the price.

Throughout its history, the Salvadorian population has always lacked the basic necessities: housing, health, nutrition, and education. Because this situation has worsened, it presents a particularly acute challenge to educators who must consciously and efficiently respond to the need for social, physical, and cultural change.

The Formation of Human Resources for Health

Faced with a reality which limits access to housing, food, education, and health for the majority of the population, in 1966, the University

---

*Note that this article was written prior to the 1992 signing of the peace treaty between the insurgency movement and the civil government.

of El Salvador (UES) rethought the formation of its programs of study and elaborated a theoretical framework to define the university as *free, democratic, humanistic,* and *popular.*

Within this theoretical framework, the UES began to rethink curriculum change toward the formation of human resources that use both the scientific method and available technologies to understand the extent and depth of the problems at hand and solve them in the service of the general population. The Faculty of Medicine, in its ten career offerings, identifies the wellness–illness continuum unique to our society as the specific objective of study. Accepting the national reality as the base, it is imperative to understand it by means of the scientific method which then becomes a necessary instrument for the contiguous socioepidemiological method.

Within the socioepidemiological focus of the wellness-illness continuum, reality is viewed as a whole, whose constant dialectical interchange results in sociohistorical contradictions. Because this historical backdrop helps to define a complex phenomenon, it requires, when referring to "health," an interdisciplinary response involving the community—the foundation of the community axis of the curriculum.

This approach to the wellness–illness continuum as a socionatural phenomenon is objective—that is, it is an observable product of men and women in their social relations and can be studied as such. Although the character of social relations is historical, with roots extending deep through the social structure, that character can be changed through human action and through dialectical relations with other phenomena and with itself. Understood in this fashion, the wellness–illness continuum is a collective phenomenon, which can be observed in the individual, and whose study would be socioepidemiological.

The socioepidemiological focus leads us to an integral, community-based study of the problems of health. Research, the study of daily problems, as the central axis of the educational process, becomes a means by which to search for an appropriate theory that orients us to formulate new proposals for the solution of problems along with the community in a particularly conscious and reflective fashion.

Current health needs are enormous; the majority of the population is living in poverty or extreme poverty. A war economy, external debt, and a budget deficit make it impossible for the state to comply with its constitutional mandate to care for the health of the population. This obligates the UES and its Faculty of Medicine to revise its curriculum and to ask this question: To whom does this curriculum respond?

In 1958, in an attempt to develop resources to support the practice of curative medicine, the Clinical Laboratory Technician program was begun in the Faculty of Medicine. In 1973, the School of Medical Technology was founded on the Leavell and Clark model and today offers nine different programs of study. A decade later, as a result of the historical analysis of the national reality of health, the curriculum was revised to address the health needs of the majority population of the country.

With the wellness–illness continuum defined as the object of study, a structural focus based on an educational model with integrated axes of study has resulted in a new educational profile: to develop professionals who will work with the population in its socionatural setting to seek solutions to its health problems and to support that population in its own transformation. The curriculum axes are developed to integrate the basic functions of the university: research, teaching, and social service. Here, research offers viable perspectives on problems in real settings while allowing alternative solutions via the scientific method and community participation.

Teaching is a process. Based on the above research, the student learns facts and develops skills and abilities to meet emerging and established health needs. Success here depends on interdisciplinary effort and community participation to find solutions by working together in the transformation of present material and spiritual conditions.

In this sense, social service provides services for and with the community, which, through the application of science and technology, modify reality and, in practice, transform the teacher, the student, and the community.

The integration of these basic functions requires a study of concrete reality and reflection upon both that reality and the study. Such integration also requires searching for an appropriate theory by which to respond to the problems revealed in practice with identified alternatives based on scientific solutions. Thus, through a spiral of knowledge and perspectives, we can begin to respond to health problems.

Basic to this model is work-study. As tasks are carried out in the institutional or community setting, problems are identified and alternative solutions for the wellness–illness continuum are presented in the settings in which they arise. This dialectic has permitted the development of an action/reflection/action model. The use of participatory research guarantees collective analyses of problems and the consolidation of critical judgments of teachers, students, and the community. It permits us to confront the realities of health by constructing a preventative-curative professional practice, with the participation of the users of institutional services and of the community.

Such alternative practice has permitted the development (with the community) of a strategy of primary health care. Inclusive to its application is a holistic vision which involves all community resources and is organized to lead to self-determination by orienting its practice to the local health system. Toward this end, efforts are made to integrate teaching and assistance. This model also obligates the faculty, through its curricular commissions, to a constant revision of the profiles of professional resources as demanded by the community, along with resultant curricular revisions in response.

Currently, efforts are underway to change the curriculum to develop an educational model that maintains as its philosophical-sociological-psychological base the health needs of the majority of the country's population. Here, the individual is seen as a product of the social structure. Social characteristics are seen in a capitalist perspective, which also encourages recognition of the need to change from individualist to societal development by making life participatory. Social changes are analyzed in the international context and the classical theoretical base is oriented toward the formation of individuals for peace.

In this regard, the curriculum involves a fundamental biophysical, chemical, and social framework based on three fundamental axes which are in constant dialectical relation to lead to the professional profile. First, the *theoretical axis* is based on the fundamentals of the natural and social sciences and identifies the wellness–illness continuum in the Salvadorian reality as the basis of the curriculum.

Second, the *methodological axis* works through the scientific method, which is applied in the epidemiological and the clinical methods in the study of the wellness–illness continuum. This teaching process leads to a critical, didactic questioning of reality that operates collectively among teachers, students, and the community.

Third, the *service axis* is the social service component of academic work in health-care institutions at different levels of complexity and in the communities. Here, the cumulative effect is to enrich social service practice generally. The model displays a vertical and a horizontal dynamic as well: in each plane intermediate skills are obtained until final training in the proposed profile.

CURRICULAR PRACTICE

In the development of the educational model for the School of Medical Technology, the real structures through which education is carried out in the faculty have been taken into account. These structures have been characterized, among other things, by: organization by department and areas of specialization which, as closed specialties, deepen knowledge in specific areas toward the ultimate formation of the specialization; the limited use of scientific investigation, weighted heavily toward natural science research methods and the absence of social research, positivist, and neo-positivist strategies which have influenced Western medical education; and, finally, the influence of the North American School—all of which have been reflected in the plan of study and programs.

Looking at the curriculum of the Faculty of Medicine from this perspective, we were obligated to find a transitional design which, despite being presented as courses, would have a logical and coherent sequential development. This would permit the development of appropriate curricular axes over time and the specific correlates necessary to provide the intermediate training relevant to concrete work and the ultimate development of the professional profile.

A very important previous step was identifying the objective of study of each of the careers offered. Depending upon the particular approach of each discipline, these will combine differently with the common objective of the entire School of Medical Technology—the wellness–illness continuum. For example, the objective of study for nursing is the wellness–illness continuum just as it is for maternal-infant health, but with an emphasis here on the maternal-infant area; for diet and nutrition, it is the wellness–illness continuum in relation to the nutritional process; for health education, it is the wellness–illness continuum in relation to the educational process. Variations, therefore, depend upon the discipline.

A second key step was the classification of each specific professional profile, which included the following: personality profile, occupational profile, and a proposal for alternative practice tied to making the resource relevant to our national reality as a support for a solution to the problems of the population. Toward this end, as a creative force, each discipline proposed an educational profile consisting of duties, activities, and in some cases specific assignments, which the trained resource should be capable of carrying out. On the other hand, if the specific career has two degree levels, bachelors and diploma, as is the case with nursing, the identification of profiles for each level is required.

Third, the question of how to design the plan of studies involved the difficulties to be found in a school which had yet to change its global academic methods. Advanced proposals by the School of Medical Technology for integrated or modular areas, for example, were not very feasible. However, in this context it was decided to use the course-work design as described at the beginning of this paper, which would orient the educational process from beginning to end.

We will identify two models in this work, the plan for a bachelors degree in nursing and in health education while taking into account two different situations: (A) nursing as a discipline with one objective of study; and (B) health education, where the objective is combined.

Situation A

In the case of the bachelor's degree in nursing, two axes and three ways of ordering courses to guide the educational process were identified: (1) the clinical axis; (2) the community axis; and (3) courses in fundamentals and methodology.

The Clinical Axis. The *clinical axis* is composed of a series of sequential courses designed to complete one part of the professional profile, in this case referring to the institutional professional profile and nursing clinic. This includes preventative-curative patient care on an individual basis but seen as part of a wider family and community context.

Throughout this axis of assignments part of the theory of the wellness–illness continuum is expounded as part of the theoretical-analytical axis. It is also given as institutional practice develops. Through teacher-assistant integration, part of the service axis is also acquired as knowledge is gained in each assignment, as well as skills, understanding, and abilities which are strengthened and integrated in the intermediate skills identified for each level.

The Community Axis. The *community axis* is formed by a series of courses under the heading of Nursing in Community Health, I–IV. Here, an experience is developed which permits both successive approximations of community health needs as well as the development of a complete program of community health in a concrete and clearly identified community, as will see. In this axis, the theory and philosophy of community work is studied in the context of a scientific, dialectic, and historical worldview, with a strong popular education component. Participatory research-action, the wellness–illness continuum at both the collective and the individual levels, and the scientific theories of sociology and anthropology are studied. Additionally, there is a work-study practicum in the community which is continuous and unique from beginning to end (lasting four academic cycles). It is in this axis that social service is carried out.

Both axes, *clinical* and *community,* are interrelated, nourishing each other in theory, practice, and methodology so that *clinical axis* courses support those of the *community axis* courses and vice versa. In this sense, learned intermediate skills are put into practice in the successive approximations of community health needs and in institutional work. This process permits the integration of knowledge, ability, and skills as well as the development of attitudes toward serving the population; the investigation of problems; the support of concrete, transformative solutions; and work with multidisciplinary teams and with the community. The process of learning is realized in the execution of a praxis in concrete reality. Again, this praxis is oriented through a continuous process of scientific investigation from beginning to end.

Courses in Fundamentals and Methodology. Courses in fundamentals and methodology involve the grouping of courses that support theory (*theoretical-analytical axis*); training (*methodology axis*); and practice (*service axis*) of the identified curricular axes.

According to the new understanding of the wellness–illness continuum and of sanitary practice as a biosocial process, we see the need to base the formation of the resource in the social and natural sciences.

In terms of social sciences, the plan of study includes a group of courses which support the theoretical-methodological base of the axes, including Elements of Sociology, Psychology, Teaching, and Educational Technology.

In terms of natural sciences, Biology, Physics, and Chemistry are studied. These support Human Biology and Microbiology which are the curricular base of the natural sciences that support the theory of the wellness–illness continuum.

In addition, a series of courses on methodology are given throughout the entire course of study, which constitute the methodological axis and whose practice is concretized in the theoretical-practical curricular axes, including: the Methodology of Scientific Investigation and Statistics, which provides the work tools for both axes; Edidemiology, which provides the methodological-theoretical component for the curricular focus and (collective) community practice; First Aid; Fundamentals of Nursing; Mental Health and Psychiatric Nursing, which complement the theory and practice of health; Administration; and English.

Situation B

In the case of health education, whose object of study combines the wellness–illness continuum and the educational process, two axes and three types of courses have also been identified: (1) the educational axis; (2) community health axis; and (3) courses of fundamentals and methodology.

The Educational Axis. *The educational axis* is made up of a series of courses whose theoretical-fundamental component is educational but whose practice is integrated into the community health axis through the practice of sanitary education at the individual level as well as at the collective, communitary, and institutional levels.

This axis develops the educational component of the *theoretical-analytical* and part of the *education methodological* component to provide the tools for concrete educational praxis, which is achieved through successive approximations based on a scientific philosophy of education. The result is a pedagological plan with emphasis on education of the adult to develop a social conscience and to achieve self-determination in the area of health. It is based on a critical didactic which applies methodologies of teaching-learning through action/reflection/action regarding problems of collective interest with an emphasis on health.

The Community Health Axis. The *community health axis* includes a series of courses which develop the theory of the wellness–illness continuum (as part of the theoretical-analytical axis) and which is developed as in the previous model (Situation A). The practicum of the educational and wellness–illness components, both institutional and community, are carried out in the social service axis. Both are integrated in successive approximations toward reality where, through practical application, they respond to that reality and by so doing allow the practical skills of the professional profile as previously outlined to be gained. At the same time, philosophical and methodological components of community work are included in this axis along with the development of skills and abilities in preventative sanitary techniques. It is worth noting that the methodology of scientific investigation serves as a tool throughout the entire axis, as it corresponds to investigation/action/participation and epidemiological methods and research. This development of sanitary praxis permits the integration of the three basic functions: teaching, research, and social service.

Courses in Fundamental and Methodology. As in the model described in Situation A, various fundamental components are identified. In terms of social sciences, the plan of study includes the same areas as in the previous model, but with a deepening and amplification through Philosophy, Sociology, Anthropology, and Psychology as related to the educational process and deepened in the educational axis.

In terms of the natural sciences, the plan of study includes the same areas as in the previous model. Various other methodology courses also support the theoretical-practical development of the curricular axes: Scientific Investigation, Statistics, English, and Administration. Both models develop through a process which moves from the general and collective toward the particular and individual, reaching a deeper understanding in the final course of study to complement the characteristic professional profile, which will be put to the test in the integrating process of social service and graduation seminar.

Practice in the Community Health Axis

As we previously established, the community health axis is developed through various courses which were designed in the corresponding syllabus as a very general theoretical project. As the experience unfolded, the programs have had to be constructed to move from practice toward theory, which has permitted increasing success through systematization of experiences. However, we have currently defined methodological strategy course programs as guides to action with this proviso: they must not become straightjackets for all programs since each experience is unique and possesses its own rhythm. Therefore, in general terms, the organization of the units of instruction has functioned as modules with objectives of transformation which, taking community work as the source of transformative objectives, have permitted the organization of theory which supports the problems to be analyzed in each unit of instruction.

Additionally, this axis promotes the development of a community health project in a specific community, with marginal communities of

San Salvadorian metropolitan areas having been selected as the target population. It should be noted that we still must expand our area of action to rural areas, which are most deficient in the formation of resources. However, urban marginal communities still retain many characteristics similar to those of rural areas; fundamentally, they are the result of the rural-urban migratory phenomenon augmented by the political-military situation.

At this time and as a goal of community work, we have worked to ensure that the community develop a process of self-determination that permits it to develop health care activities through its own organization and conscious participation. In the process, health personnel act as facilitators or catalysts rather than as community leaders as has been proposed on occasion. Additionally, health personnel have a specific technical role to carry out depending on their areas of specialization which, again, must be put in the service of the expressed and real needs of the community so that health care personnel can participate in the successful transformation of a community's health.

Another element to be taken into account here is this: the wellness–illness continuum is a socionatural product. This implies the integral whole of the life of the community as a product of all its social activity, and additionally the genetic possibilities each individual represents. Taken together, these interacting conditions result in the maintenance or loss of health throughout life.

In the search for and resolution of problems, community health intervention proposals to be developed must take into account possibilities inherent in the community itself. In many cases, the community has access to resources offered by different institutions and organizations which are not efficiently used. Through a process of community self-determination, these resources could be used to successfully carry out development projects to improve morbi-mortality profiles while keeping in mind that base causal elements are the result of general structural problems which, if not modified, will limit the reach of community health programs.

Thus, in terms of the problem of work in the community, the following developmental steps can be identified:

1. Immersion and Integration: In this phase, the teacher-student research team approaches the community in a real, physical way. This is initiated by the selection process itself and continues with a recognition of its geography and infrastructure by an initial contact with the organizations and population of the community. In this context, the approach to immediately identifiable spiritual aspects must be progressively deepened, which implies a greater interaction with and reinforcement of community organizations as well as increased interaction with the community's needs, hopes, and visions of the world. This process of

integration is carried out through interaction and participatory reflection between the research team and the community.

2. Identification of Health Needs: In this phase, a diagnosis of health needs is carried out. This diagnosis is the product of transversal epidemiological investigation using participatory investigation/action methodology in which the research group is widened with the participation of students, teachers, and members of the community who share in the planning, execution, and reflection of the results obtained.

3. Prioritization of Problems: As key to the development of the community health program, the team and community together analyze and reflect on the results of the diagnosis. With the help of the team, the community prioritizes problems and determines which problems will be dealt with through community action.

4. Programming: The work plan must allow for consideration of the health actions to be developed during the entire time the team will be in the community and for combining the skills the students gain over time, the resources of the community, and those of the UES.

5. Development of Community or Participatory Projects: Through this concrete work, the organizations of the community, its skills, and self-determination are reinforced.

6. Evaluation of the Process: Evaluation must proceed by participation. Currently, we have succeeded in developing a process of participatory evaluation which looks at each work-product at the level of the teaching-learning process. We have been able to evaluate community projects together with the community but have not yet been able to introduce the community element into the evaluation of the student during the entire process.

7. Coordination: The coordination and cooperation of the many organizations participating in the community work is a fundamental component of the process. Coordination is carried out at the community (local) level, at the institutional level, and at the intra-university level. Additionally, this coordination must take into account that community work and community health can only be carried out efficiently by multidisciplinary teams with democratic and equal participation.

Strategic Elements in the Implementation of the Curricular Change

In terms of the planning processes, it is intended that all careers in the School of Medical Technology progressively participate in the curricular change and with flexibility implement all informal structures in a transition phase to facilitate the process of curricular planning. This will permit the maintenance of a dynamic development that, without being disordered, will offer freedom for each teaching team relative to its own process of theoretical-practical development and creativity in building its curricular proposal. This planning is seen in two levels:

1. Careers: Curricular subcommissions have been re-created in each of the careers offered. These include teachers from that career (students are not yet incorporated) who move forward, coordinate, and direct the curricular planning process within the career. However, planning should encourage the global participation of the teaching collective and those involved in generalizing the goals of curricular change. These subcommissions should present new curriculum proposals to the curricular commission of the School of Medical Technology and, with the support of the teaching personnel, should explain and justify the proposals, subsequently incorporating into their proposal relevant observation of the curricular commission.

2. The School of Medical Technology: The curricular commission of the School was formed in 1985. It is made up of the director and one teacher from each career, the directorate of the school, and the members of the community health unit. The goal was the formation of the multidisciplinary team to orient and direct the curricular change of the School of Medical Technology.

This commission has worked to elaborate a new general philosophical-scientific-methodological framework as the theoretical framework and reference point for all curricular proposals of the school, assuming the educational model already described. Additionally, it discusses the preliminary curricular proposals of each career subcommission. After successive drafts, the proposals are fit into the general framework and the project is then approved. The commission has also established a process for training and assistance in curricular planning. In terms of legal assistance, the curricular project is submitted for the analysis and approval of the legal body of the faculty and university.

Implementation of Curricular Change

The process of curricular change, while difficult and delicate, has been essential. The teaching staff at the University of El Salvador and its Medical School, with 150 years of traditional medical formation, has accepted the doctor as the only and "inherent leader" of the health team. In this "doctor-centered" view, careers in the School of Medical

Technology have been seen as "paramedic," in other words, secondary or complementary to the work of the doctor. The new curriculum proposal of the School of Medical Technology, which included new roles and profiles aimed toward integrating and broadening the traditional health team, is based on a wellness–illness global plan, involving health needs and their solutions. From there began the obstacles and misunderstandings of the new curricular proposal.

To this must be added the general scarcity of human, material, and financial resources which limit the School of Medical Technology within the Faculty of Medicine. In this process, we want to highlight the following aspects which have been key in the implementation process.

Logistics

The School of Medical Technology was born in 1973 without its own budget although the larger budget of the Faculty of Medicine was increased. Currently, the school still does not have its own budget. Compounding this structural problem were the cries against the closings and ransackings that the university has suffered over the past 15 years, during which its sudden closing in 1980 was the most dramatic.

Despite this, the School of Medical Technology has succeeded in implementing 90 percent of its career plan due to student support as well as international and specific project donations. It is worth noting that currently 60 percent of the careers offered have one or more projects financed with international aid—the possibility of more aid exists because of the vibrancy of the careers themselves. Also, a teacher-service strategy has been advanced which permits the use of extra-university infrastructure and equipment (especially for careers such as anesthesia and radiotechnology).

Those careers with new curricular proposals have also developed their own community resources to implement the community axis. This has been possible specifically because of the method of participatory research that has been developed.

Teacher Training

Teacher training is another important area which has been developed parallel to the planning, implementation, and execution of the new curriculum. Training methods have been varied and have ranged from continuous training in the process of teaching to short one-and-two-week courses between cycles offered to all teachers, as well as training courses outside the School of Medical Technology in the UES and the exterior. Basic themes to support curricular development have included: scientific methodology; socio-philosophical framework; pedagogy; curricular design; epidemiology; the process of the wellness–illness continuum; and other specific areas. The school has used its own financing and external financing for this area; however, the process continues and the need still exists for a systematic deepening of training.

New Support Structures

In the implementation process, the need to develop new support structures became clear. Some have been temporary such as special commissions of teachers from various careers to respond to concrete problems in areas of common study, both in the larger context of the UES or within the school itself, for example, with difficult courses like Human Biology, Special Chemistry course, General Psychology, Research, General Disease, Classification, Graduate Seminar, Social Services, and so on.

Another structure created toward this end is the community health unit whose principle function is to make the community health axis a viable component of the new curriculum. The unit coordinates and integrates this component to support work within multidisciplinary teams while maintaining a coherence of focus toward the community. Support for this process comes through the integration of teaching, research, and social service.

The community health unit has functioned both directly in teaching, in teacher-student assistance, in support of the curricular plan as well as in teacher training. It has also aided in the integration of theoretical elements resulting from the analysis and reflection of specific practice toward establishing general guidelines in the development of community work and community health and in achieving goals and objectives. Its resources—scarce relative to the ever-increasing demand of the new curriculum—are multidisciplinary, with experience in social process and in the wellness–illness continuum for an epidemiolic and participation-action research perspective. Important here as well is the use of expertise specific to its own career profile. Resources are lacking in such areas as social psychology, philosophy, economics, and pedagogy—all of which complete the global vision of the socionatural reality of health in Salvadorian communities.

Coordination with Other Units

A strategy of developing coordination among multiple areas and sectors must be included in the process of developing a new curricular focus. Coordination must be established with various levels and grades such as:

1. First level: among the various careers that make up the School of Medical Technology.
2. Second level: with the Faculty of Medicine and with units of administrative support such as Academic Administration, the Office of the Dean, Planning, etc.
3. Third level: with intra-university faculties and central units.
4. Fourth level: extra-university with other state and private institutions.
5. Fifth level: with international organizations for teaching and technical cooperation such as PASO, INCAP, international universities, etc.
6. Sixth level: with the communities in which the community axis is carried out.

Working in Teams

The traditional approach in health has been individualistic, isolated, and fragmented. It is fundamental to develop a new educational and professional practice from the perspective of working in teams, trying to identify members of equal importance and participation in concrete, integrating work in order to transform reality. In the conception of *team*, there can be various levels of development:

1. First level: multidisciplinary teams with the participation of diverse disciplines.
2. Second level: inter-sector teams with the participation of students, teachers, and administrative personnel.
3. Third level: teacher-student and community teams, integrating the university and the community in the same work—in other words, external and internal agents in the community.

This process makes us reflect more deeply about the goal of changing attitudes, ideology, and interpretations of reality as well as the need to continue a process of self-criticism.

Administration of Curriculum

Administration of curriculum refers to the form in which the planning, organization, implementation, evaluation, and supervision of the process of curricular development is carried out by all participants. The actions of those with leadership positions is emphasized; they must understand the curricular proposal in all its historic, political, philosophical, pedagogical, and methodological dimensions and share it—both the workings of the educational model in all its detail and the professional practice to be obtained by it. Only a broad understanding of all of these aspects would permit the adequate development of the curricular process both at the level of career and school.

On the other hand, it is the teachers who will actively carry out the curriculum and the students who will be the subjects of that activity. All should know and reflect deeply on its successes and goals both in its design and functioning. All should analyze current successes and limitations to carry out constructive self-criticism of their participation in the process to enrich and improve it dynamically.

LIMITATIONS FOR THE CURRICULAR TRANSFORMATION OF THE SCHOOL OF MEDICAL TECHNOLOGY

The development of the new curricular plan, however unique or appealing, is plagued with dangers. It comes up against academic, administrative, political, and student limitations.

Academic Limitations

University reform and one of its expressions—curricular transformation—is still not seen as fundamental necessity in our university. In general terms, curricular designs in the UES are based on a course structure, so that knowledge is given in a fragmented manner with the expectation that by the end of the curriculum all students have integrated their knowledge. This results in the formation of human resources that cannot confront the problem we have put forth—the unique and complete reality. Those teaching units that administer the curriculum are departments whose vertical training and isolation are well known and that do not favor change.

Looking more deeply at the academic problem, we encounter at the Faculty of Medicine the method of transmission of understanding of subject matter. Here, the basis of teaching is the classroom and tutorial practice, usually hospital oriented. As previously described, the departments, formed around distinct specialities, are those responsible for the teachers and their method of teaching. In many cases, as well, departments are divided by subspecialties which involve repetition of theories that are externally elaborated and, thus, isolated.

To date, the study of the wellness–illness continuum is not integrated or based on a diagnosis of Salvadorian reality. Although the official documents which describe the objectives seem theoretically well-elaborated, in practice they are not carried out, resulting in the formation of human resources that are detached from reality. All of this can be seen in the School of Medical Technology—the changes which have been made do not have deep logistical, administrative, library, or academic support. In this sense, we can look at other examples. Human Biology as a course made up of three components—anatomy, physiology, and biochemistry—is a curricular component that needs more integration in practice to reinforce theory and, at the same time, more theory to compliment practice. It is also necessary to use the library for certain objectives. Yet, because the conception and methodology of teaching have not changed, a high rate of failure (88% in Cycle 2 89/90) has resulted, decimating the student population. This phenomenon is repeated in courses such as General Physics, General Biology, and Special Chemistry also resulting in student desertion.

Social science fundamentals are served by other departments that do not satisfy the objectives proposed in the new curriculum—general philosophy, sociology, and teaching—and we find ourselves obligated to ask for help from teachers of those departments at the school for its specific development. Although this practice has given some favorable results, such is not always possible given the lack of resources. Nor should this practice be seen as an appropriate response to the prevailing problems. Without integration into the educational project at hand, borrowings from other departments can only serve as a stop gap or preparatory measure. The School of Medical Technology has grown because of increased student demand—for which needs are always greater. Adding this to the new focus, we are continuously confronted with trained and untrained teachers and students which result in a constant disequilibrium, lending itself to different interpretations of the curriculum as well as negative attitudes toward its implementation. The development of careers is not uniform. There is a deficiency in the number of human resources which results in exhausting academic workloads that do not leave the time necessary for deeper reflection and enrichment of the curricular process. This results in a slow process of change because of inefficient student, teacher, and administrative participation. Active and conscious participation by all is a necessity. Participation is fundamental and must be continuous.

Administrative Limitations

Because of a rigid administrative structure, the support necessary for a more flexible curriculum does not readily exist. For the most part, the structure is oriented toward the Faculty of Medicine. Although efforts have been made to establish more adequate coordination between the schools, it has not yet been possible. Criteria for recognizing the role of the resources that form the School of Medical Technology are lacking, resulting in those resources still being considered as "paramedics." A process must be developed that would make the various career profiles compatible. Teamwork is essential here as resources confront the problems specific to their areas of expertise.

To this date, as well, administrative personnel are not efficiently incorporated into the process of curricular change and are not taken into account as a participating element in the formation of the student.

Regarding the label, "paramedic careers," we must explain again that the School of Medical Technology is made up on nine disciplines, the majority of which form complete resources not to assist the doctor but with a focus toward public health which integrates with the doctor into a health team where each resource has a specific profile of development, where leadership can be held by any member of the team, and all act in a coordinated manner in response to the wellness–illness continuum. We are convinced that as long as the problem is not confronted with an epidemiological and public health focus we will continue in efforts that are not integrated, not coordinated, and that duplicate work. The resulting impact on the health of the population will not be significant.

Political Limitations

Accepting as politics the general guidelines of the work of the school, we can analyze the life of the School of Medical Technology. In the School of Medical Technology no structural changes have taken place. For example, the existing rules are obsolete; of 12 specific objectives of the school, 11 refer to the doctor, and only one to the "paramedic."

The last five years, however, have seen fundamental changes in university rules, philosophical ideas, and identification of basic functions. Such changes have still to be incorporated into the rules governing the School of Medicine and its daily practice. The new focus of the School of Medical Technology, which is compatible with the fundamental changes just mentioned, also causes problems in the execution of the new curriculum.

We can analyze some of the multiple problems generated by this situation. As previously explained, the School of Medical Technology administers nine careers which, translated into a high and growing student, teacher, and administrative population, results in an increasing need to have its own continuous representation in the governing university bodies: teaching, student, and administrative. In order to do so, there must be changes in the legal basis of the School of Medicine.

The hegemonic group that characterizes only teachers of the School of Medicine constantly deny the right of the professors of the School of

Medical Technology to execute an electoral function, which, according to Article 24 of the University Code, is interpreted as prejudicial to the school. Of 23 professors, only 11 are recognized. In addition and despite an existing code regulating the teaching function, the commission created to implement the code is coordinated by the School of Medicine.

In our view, the commission is not interested in performing its function, which has resulted in a considerable backlog in the classification of new teachers and still more in the re-classification of more senior faculty. If the process were streamlined, we would have approximately 40 professors with the right to participate in the governing bodies of the school. However, we note that in the School of Medicine, when administrative teaching posts are assigned, democratic procedures are not followed as described in the University Code.

Student Limitations

The student component, considered as the objective of teaching, is not organized and is not effectively incorporated into the process of curricular change. While the first steps are just being taken to resolve this situation, neither are the students sufficiently represented in the governing bodies of the School of Medical Technology nor in the School of Medicine.

It is worthwhile to ask this question: In spite of what has been described, *is* the School of Medical Technology stagnant? The answer is *no*.

The politics of democratization now being pushed in the University of El Salvador are creating a gap in relation to the nondemocratization of the Faculty of Medicine. Currently, however, the majority of personnel of the School of Medical Technology are aware of the curricular changes proposed based on university reform and as the university's particular answer to the problems of health in the country.

22

Here There Be Dragons: Departing the Behaviorist Paradigm for State Board Regulation*

Julia E. Gould and Em Olivia Bevis

*A*ncient mariners seldom ventured far from the shores of the known world. Rare exceptions occurred: isolated, generally unrecorded voyages, the pilot books that did not become guides for others. Intrepid Northmen found their way to Greenland and then on to North America, star-led Polynesians peopled the far-flung islands of the Pacific, and the papyrus-shipped Phoenicians rode the currents to Central America. For the most part, the Chinese, Japanese, Indians, and Europeans hugged the shore.

Old cartographers drew clumsy charts of the known world. Out from the coasts, away from the easy passages in the deep and unknown ocean, fierce-looking reptiles were drawn with great Gothic letters warning "HERE THERE BE DRAGONS." Everyone knew that dragons were not the only danger facing sailors foolish enough to challenge the deep. Other monsters lurked there. As one neared the equator the waters boiled, heating the pitch with which the ships were caulked, melting it and allowing the sea to swamp and sink the ships. Last, but just as deadly, somewhere out there was the end of the world, and unwary ships sailed over the brink and were lost forever to heaven and to loved ones.

---

*Gould, J. E., & Bevis, E. O. (1992). Here there be dragons: Departing the behaviorist paradigm for state board regulation. *Nursing & Health Care, 13*(3), 126–133. © National League for Nursing.

This metaphor serves well for current events in nursing education where huge changes are occurring. The familiar behaviorist shoreline charts only philosophies, conceptual frameworks, concepts and theories, behavioral objectives, and objectives-driven evaluation. The vast new world of critical thinking, emancipation, reality-based-phenomenological learning, creativity, and committed caring-community-connectedness lies over the uncharted seas in which "there be dragons." These dragons could endanger the ship of nursing education and ultimately nursing and health care itself. Yet, if we do not explore the unknown, what vast wealth are we foregoing? It is proposed here that brave and intelligent educators can engage in carefully plotting a course, drawing maps, and keeping pilot books, thereby skillfully devising criteria or quality controls. With these tools, educators can defy the myths of dragons and explore new worlds and new paths to the "East" with the spices, silks, and gold that are the true treasures of critical consciousness, praxis, emancipation, critical thinking, caring, and community connectedness. These treasures have the potential of making nursing a moral force for change in the health care system and in the world.

THE CURRENT REGULATORY PARADIGM

The current regulatory paradigm is derived from the traditional educational paradigm, which is behaviorist. The behaviorist curriculum model, as proposed by Tyler (1949), was first tried in nursing education in 1954 (Sand, 1955) at the University of Washington in Seattle. Ole Sand, employed by that school to direct a project to improve the nursing curriculum, engaged Ralph Tyler as consultant. The result was not only a new curriculum but a book that became a popular guide for curriculum and the basis for graduate courses in curriculum construction across the nation. Nursing education experienced a rapid paradigm shift to the behaviorist Tylerian paradigm. This paradigm, as used in nursing education, was influenced by Mager (1962) to be hard-core behaviorist and adapted as a prototype for nursing by Bevis (1973). Bevis prescribed the following products of curriculum development as necessary to the approvable and accreditable curriculum (1988): philosophy; conceptual framework (concepts, theories, or threads); program, course, and level objectives; learning activity, modular, or unit objectives; objectives-driven, detailed content outlines; objectives-driven evaluation; and classroom and clinical activities.

The behaviorist paradigm has further attributes that are expected to appear in the written plan or are assumed by faculty and usually followed by them. Not all of these attributes are related to behaviorism; many are simply traditional and connected to the behaviorist curriculum by custom, convention, and practice.

1. *A detailed list of content including every aspect of nursing and medicine that is to be taught in class* has resulted in an attempt to "teacher proof" the curriculum and make it content-driven without attention to the current realities of practice. This causes teacher anxiety that inhibits any departure from the content list, curtails individual teacher creativity, and diminishes the class's ability to move with the emerging content of student experiences. It also reduces the importance of educative teaching-learning activities, such as creativity, critical thinking, pattern recognition, meaning making, significance appreciation, and developing insights.

2. *An assumption that reliance on lecture is the most effective and efficient method of teaching* has resulted in dependence on passive learning methods that research demonstrates is ineffective, in that all but 10% of what is learned is forgotten in 2 years' time. Lecture is also ineffective in teaching crucial intellectual and moral capabilities. The characteristics of an educated person are among these and include: critical thinking; creativity; flexibility; emancipation from oppressive and/or conformitive thinking; critical social consciousness; caring; ethical and moral commitment; insights; foresight; anticipatory inventiveness; originality; flexible strategizing; style; personal power, its acquisition, use, and sharing; a sense of the significant; ability to cut cleanly to the core of issues; vision of the assumptions underlying issues and the assumptions underlying assumptions; ability to engage in dialogue rather than polemics; skilled use of intuition; commitment to fraternal/sororal colleagueship/friendship; a sense of social/professional/personal responsibility; a continuing search for meaning; and a sense of community connectedness and commitment.

3. *An assumption that the teacher is the authority and the students know little or nothing* leads to received knowledge and to passive acceptance on the part of students that "teacher knows best" and that they have little or nothing to learn from each other or from nurses in practice. In a covert way, it teaches students to be dominated easily, to maintain the status quo, and to accept the discount of being driven by a curriculum they had no part in developing and no modalities for steering. It participates in making students immature with a desire to be "spoon-fed."

4. *An assumption that the classroom is where one learns "theory" and clinical areas are where one "applies" theory* leads to the inevitable confusion that classroom content is based in reality and that reality resembles what one learns in the classroom. Nursing practice is shunned as the basis for nursing education, which causes a schism. It can lead to the assumption that reality may be damaging to the student's health, and is to be avoided, and also to

the myth that with proper instruction new graduates can change reality. Inexorably, education becomes isolated in some sort of a dream fog. An obvious logic that all practice fields, to be optimally effective, must be based in the realities of their practice is ignored. Benner (1984) has addressed this point.

5. *An assumption exists that nurses in practice generally are poor role models, do not "keep up," expect the wrong things of new graduates, and are antagonistic to educators and to nursing education's goals.* The subassumption is that education can make the necessary changes in nursing education and practice, in the sick-care system, and ultimately in the world political and social order as it affects health, without the alliance of their colleagues in practice. The flaw in this assumption is that it ignores the society of caregivers who must forge alliances in order to form a more equitable and responsive health care system. It also robs students of the beneficial influence, expertise, and experiences of the largest segment of nurses, the nurses in practice.

6. *An assumption that all learning is defined as a change in behaviors that are derived from teacher-defined objectives* leads to objectives-driven evaluation, so that only those behaviors identified by faculty as valuable will be seen as meriting credit toward success. The error in this is that all other things learned are treated as unnecessary, irrelevant, tangential, worthless, or even detrimental.

SETTING THE PARADIGM IN CONCRETE

The current paradigm and its assumptions, though once very helpful to nursing, have become pernicious and injurious to nursing as a whole. Tyler has become, not just a guide for curriculum development, but a legal code that, through nurse practice acts and their rules regulating nursing education, dictates not quality, as was intended, but the whole process of teaching nursing. Tyler's curriculum development products have been translated into essential components, without evidence of which, state board approval may be compromised. If approval was withdrawn from a program, its graduates would not be allowed to take the licensing examination. That is institutionalization at its most powerful.

SETTING A COURSE

What this tells us is that no paradigm, no one curriculum development model, can be allowed to dominate state board attempts to regulate nursing education and ensure quality. Regulation should assess quality, not dictate models or paradigms. Columbus thought he was seeking a route east to the Indies, a new route to bring the riches and spices of India to Europe. What he found was entirely different, but on embarking he knew what he sought. Following that simile, what is sought here is a way to assess quality and to ensure public safety, without dictating the curriculum model. Georgia seeks to regulate while providing flexibility and choices in old and new curriculum paradigms.

THE CONTEXT AND HISTORY OF CHANGE

Context. During 1990, the Georgia Board of Nursing adopted new educational rules that departed from the behaviorist paradigm. Three main players were significant in their development, the first being site visits and the insights gained there.

According to the rules regulating nursing education in Georgia, the Board of Nursing representatives conduct site visits to nursing education programs to verify compliance. Two to three-day site visits to the 37 registered nurse programs are conducted routinely every 4 years to regulate them and ensure quality. Visits are also made to programs that are developing, have documented noncompliance, have a new dean/director, and/or have a major curriculum revision.

The Board staff includes a nursing education consultant who participates with a designated Board member to make these visits. The education consultant also provides consultative assistance to programs requesting help with educational goals or problems.

A second player was the Board's Education Committee. This committee is comprised of approximately 20 people: educators representing associate degree, diploma, and baccalaureate nursing programs from public and private institutions; nursing service representatives; a Board member liaison; and the nursing education consultant. At the direction of the Board, the committee reviews and/or drafts educational rules, considers matters pertaining to education, and plans the annual meeting of deans and directors.

The third player was the annual meeting of deans and directors, at which information is shared from the Board and from the National Council of State Boards of Nursing. Ideas, issues, and other items of mutual concern are also discussed and sometimes referred to the Education Committee.

History. During 1988–1989, a persistent topic of conversation during site visits, in the Education Committee, and at the annual meeting of deans and directors, was faculty workload or, more aptly, faculty overload. It became apparent through these discussions that faculty were taking a serious look not only at the way in which they spent their time, but also at the quality of that time, its effectiveness in educating students, and its energizing or, as was often the case, enervating effects. Efforts to amend nursing faculty workloads at the administrative level of parent institutions were time-consuming and fruitless. Faculty spent hours accumulating data to justify all aspects of a change in workload only to be told, in the final analysis, that they were consistent with the parent institution's workload expectations. Of course, the matter had a basis in economics and politics. Under the cloud of the workload issue, students focused heavily on time and stress as the significant variables in the learning process. Learning, under these conditions, took a back seat to survival. Faculty who were evaluating the quality and cost-effectiveness of the way their time was spent were realizing that, while they could not change the position of the parent institution's administration, they could take a different tack by selecting more meaningful learning activities within the given time frame and within selected settings. In other words, they had a choice about the quality of time expended. One emerging insight was that stress was a response to several variables. In this case, a significant causal variable was the catalog of specific content prescribed for each course. Attempts to improve quality and to control the educational productivity of time were at odds with the faculty's commitment to the prescribed, detailed, content outline.

During the 1989–1990 school year, Board visitors, stimulated by faculty and student concerns and the workshops and literature about the new nursing educational paradigms, began to enter into different kinds of discussions with faculty during the scheduled site visits. The usual routine on the first day had been that the visitors reviewed requested program materials. On the second day, faculty were asked to share their ideas about the strengths of the program and any planned changes or to clarify points raised by the visitors. During the 1989–1990 term, faculty were asked to describe classroom and clinical learning activities that helped the written course materials come alive. The change in insights provided to the site visitors, and often to faculty, was a revelation. Faculty cohesiveness, creativity, and energy, or lack of it, were immediately apparent. If faculty and students were engaging in creative learning activities, faculty were very quick to describe them, to urge a colleague to describe one, and to give credit to one another. A rehabilitation course that seemed dry and repetitive in print was full of a variety of creative and educative learning activities when described verbally; for example, students simulated limited mobility and negotiated the highways and byways of the local shopping mall. Conversely, faculty who were oriented toward passive learning in their teaching stated that their classroom learning activities consisted only of lecture and discussion.

Impetus toward drafting educational rules that were more flexible was triggered by the passage of the revised Georgia Registered Professional Nurse Practice Act in April 1990. A logical and necessary consequence of this was to review all the Board's rules to ensure that they were consistent with the new statute. The educational rules underwent a major overhaul in 1984. Minor revisions had been adopted in the interim but it was now appropriate for an examination of all rules. This task fell to the Education Committee. Concomitantly, interest had been increasing in the emerging paradigms in nursing education that departed the traditional behaviorist models. The committee was becoming aware that the educational rules did not permit any departure from the traditional behaviorist products of curriculum development.

The nursing education consultant who staffs the committee, prepared a working draft of the new rules to expedite the committee's work. The work sessions were stimulating, productive, and exciting. The committee decided to overhaul the rules to provide flexibility for faculty and students who were moving away from the behaviorist model while enabling those who wished to maintain the status quo to do so.

THE NEW RULES

Because it would be impossible to describe all of the rule changes, only a few that are illustrative will be compared and discussed.

The rules regarding curriculum and faculty received the most attention. Georgia was set on a course of allowing and promoting curricula that facilitate the graduation of a better-educated nurse. Three old rules, in the behaviorist mode, were merged into one streamlined rule.

The old rule stated that (the curriculum shall be):

- Developed by faculty to reflect the philosophy, program objectives, and rationale for its organization and development in keeping with accepted past and present socioeconomic, educational, and nursing standards and trends;
- Developed so that objectives, course content, and learning activities demonstrate a clear relationship to each other.
- Objectives shall be measurable and feasible, and serve as a basis for course development and evaluation of students.

The new rule states that (the curriculum shall be)

- Developed by faculty so that the philosophy or list of assumptions, learning goals, written plan for its organization and development, teaching/learning strategies, and critique of learning are internally consistent.

The old rule statement about standards and trends was revised to stand as a separate rule.

The old rules prescribed that a curriculum must have a philosophy. The new rule permits the option of not having a philosophy, per se, but of having assumptions either in a group or scattered throughout the program; for example, for each course, for policies, or for clinical learning activities.

The old rules stated that objectives must be attainable and feasible in ways that could be assessed behaviorally. They required that objectives, content, and learning activities be related to each other. Further, course development and student evaluation must be based on objectives. All of this is consistent with behaviorist curriculum theory.

The new rule substitutes learning goals for objectives. Objectives, in nursing education, connote hard-line behaviorism. According to collective tradition, arising out of Mager, each objective must include only one measurable, feasible behavior. The term "learning goals" has no such accessories or appendages. It equates to Dewey's "ends-in-view" in that goals provide intent and direction for movement allowing one to be content if proceeding in an imprecise, inexact, and uncertain way toward a general aim. Goals allow for ambiguity; objectives, as used in nursing education, dictate specificity.

The old rules included the requirement for a rationale for curricular organization and development that evolved in 1988 when the term conceptual framework was deleted. The written plan, in the new rule, is more paradigm inclusive paradigms. Faculty can portray this plan as a narrative, an outline, a table, a diagram, or as a combination as long as the organization and development of the curriculum is systematically and clearly described. Note that no course content outline is required.

The requirement that evaluation be objectives driven has been supplanted by one of critique of learning. The shift from evaluation to critique is an ideological and practical one. Critique can include evaluation, yet it presupposes a different relationship between faculty and students. Criticism, according to Stenhouse (1975) and Bevis and Watson (1989), means a participatory determination of appropriateness and progress among students and faculty. Criticism rests not in authority, as does evaluation, but in trust, in a valuing of excellence of scholarship, and in a mutual desire to improve and grow. Evaluation, as it is traditionally used, is rooted in some real or imagined authority or in the faculty's accepted version of truth or rightness—usually called "objectively held criteria." For some schools of thought, what behaviorism has never satisfactorily dealt with are characteristics and learnings such as critical thinking, creativity, meaning, and caring. The paradigm shift in nursing education, and the subsequent shift in Board rules, are designed to enable emancipatory and educative curricula that are geared to critical thinking, creativity, meaning making, and caring to find legitimate curriculum expression.

The intent of the three old rules was that the curriculum was to have uniform elements, traceably related to each other, according to accepted formulas (Mager or Bevis, e.g.). The purpose was internal consistency. The former rules dictated that required components, have a clear relationship. The new rule does require components but these are stated more broadly and describe the quality of the relationship of the components. It is suggestive of a curriculum that shows a logical, sequential, cohesive progression within the paradigm or paradigms being used.

Another rule change that reflects a significant shift in approach is the following one.

The old rule stated that (the curriculum shall be)

- inclusive of classroom and clinical instruction in the use of the nursing process with patients/clients throughout the life span who are experiencing common physical and mental health problems and illnesses, incorporating promotion and maintenance of health.

The new rule states that (the curriculum shall be)

- inclusive of classroom and clinical learning activities using the nursing process/problem-solving and emphasizing creativity and critical thinking in reality-based nursing situations with people of all age groups with commonly occurring acute and long-term physical and mental health problems, illnesses, and experiences incorporating promotion and maintenance of health.

The revised rule substituted the interactive phrase "learning activities" for the unidimensional word "instruction." Instruction, according to Bevis (Bevis & Watson, 1989), is telling—providing with information. It implies received knowledge, authority vested in the program's accepted version of truth, and passive learning—listening, taking notes, memorizing content and directions on how to do procedures. The term "classroom and clinical learning activities" connotes active learning, learner participation, shared power, or student/teacher empowerment, and communicates a "doing learning" by direct participation involving both teachers and students.

The framers of the new rules thought nursing process rather linear in structure and mechanical in its effect but felt that it was too entrenched in nursing at this time to mount its successful removal from the rules, though it does represent a paradigm prescription. Thinking to provide some flexibility, they added "problem-solving." At least with that as an alternative, one can construe that there are a variety of ways to go about examining issues and problems and that approach and methodology can be the choice of the faculty or students. Nursing process has come to have specific meanings with set subprocesses that occur in some predetermined sequence.

The emphasis on creativity and critical thinking reflects the Board's belief as to how essential these intellectual skills are to the ability to practice nursing effectively in the current, complex health care system.

The addition of "in reality-based nursing situations" reflects a belief that nursing is a practice field and as such should be taught in ways that base it in the realities of the common, day-to-day practice of nursing.

The rules governing the selection or development of learning activities were given a slant quite different from the previous rule.

The old rule stated that

- the nursing education program shall provide clinical learning experiences in a variety of settings to meet the objectives of each course with a clinical component.

The new rule states that

- the methods/criteria/strategies used to select and critique classroom and clinical learning activities and teacher/student interactions, which are congruent with the learning goals of the curriculum, shall be documented in writing.

The repealed rule again forces a tie-in of objectives with the clinical learning experiences that *shall* be provided by the educational program. Thus, the possibilities of student participation in their selection is omitted and a rationale of behaviorist logic is assumed. The new rule expands curriculum development paradigm choices by simply asking for a written description of the methods used to select and critique them. The rule still attempts to provide for internal consistency amongst the goals, learning activities, and teacher/student interactions. The emphasis on the nursing program providing learning experiences is shifted to describing what is seen by faculty as desirable education. It focuses on two things, the type of teacher/student interactions that the faculty believes facilitates the best learning and the learning activities.

The fact that faculty have to document in writing necessitates systematic thinking about the curriculum and committing those ideas and/or practices to paper that were already in place, in many instances, and that faculty verbalize. This documentation of the criteria used to select learning activities and teacher/student interactions shifts the emphasis from lists of content to the real, daily-occurring curriculum of the classroom and clinical area. It demonstrates that it is really what students are experiencing, in clinical situations and in interactions with faculty, that contain both the legitimate, the illegitimate, and the hidden curriculum. It forces some introspection by faculty and students about what kinds of learning activities and what kinds of teacher/student interactions are most geared to certain types of learning. This is a significant shift in allowing faculties and students options for paradigms. The documentation can show that those learning activities are chosen that have the best chance of enabling students to learn faculty preselected and prescribed content outlines, or it can show something to the effect that "those learning activities are chosen that students, faculty, and staff think will help the student learn to be self-directed . . . etc." (Murray, 1989).

Another aspect of the above new rule, which is closely related, is the next one.

The former rule stated that

- faculty shall select clinical learning experiences in collaboration with agency personnel.

The new rule states that

- clinical learning activities, selected collaboratively by faculty, agency personnel, and students (if applicable) shall occur in a variety of settings.

The switch here is from a rule that excludes students in the decision-making process regarding their own educational needs to one that includes them if the faculty deem it is appropriate. It sets a precedent of making it rule-possible to share power collaboratively with students. It keeps the valuable and necessary tie with practice people and actively encourages a collaborative process in the selection of learning activities in "reality-based nursing situations" referred to earlier. This is paradigm related but in a permissive rather than a restrictive way. It decreases the usual restrictions and opens the rules to more flexibility, creativity, and critical thinking for teachers, students, and agency personnel.

In the new rules, evaluation took a decided turn. The old and new rules contrast to show this.

The old rules stated

- clinical performance evaluation shall be designed to measure competence through the demonstration of skills and ability to apply the nursing process.
- written examinations shall test for various levels of learning with emphasis on application of the nursing process.

The new rule states

- the methods/criteria/strategies used to critique/evaluate student learning and progress, which are congruent with the learning goals of the curriculum, shall be documented in writing.

The old rules, consistent with the behaviorist model, emphasized measurement, demonstration of skills, and the ability to apply the nursing process. They also prescribed written tests that would focus on the nursing process. The new rule focuses on the process of critiquing and evaluating while maintaining internal consistency. Flexibility for faculty and students to use a variety of options, rather than previously prescribed ones, is provided.

The rules concerning faculty qualifications were revised to shift the focus from flat, content-driven credentials to a description of faculty preparation and expertise consistent with learning goals.

The old rules stated that

- a nursing education program shall employ faculty with graduate preparation and experience in the following nursing areas: adult health; maternal-infant health; child health; mental health; and community health (for a baccalaureate program);
- a faculty member shall have clinical qualifications in the area in which she/he serves as an instructor.

The new rule states that

- a nursing education program shall employ faculty with graduate preparation and expertise necessary to enable the learning goals of the curriculum.

The Board requires each faculty member to submit a Faculty Qualification Record as part of the program's annual report. The responses to the new questions have yielded a kaleidoscope of rich descriptions of academic credentials, practice, community service, and topics of particular interest. They give new meaning to the term "faculty qualifications."

SITE VISIT CHANGES

The new rules lead to changes in the way that site visits were conducted during 1990–1991. Subsequent to an initial meeting with the dean/director, the visitors met with faculty before any review of written program materials took place. Faculty were asked to describe classroom and clinical learning activities, which emphasized creativity and critical thinking, in each of their courses. Teacher/student interactions were also shared.

The site visits had a new excitement that demonstrated a collegial-participatory relationship between the Board and the program. Learning activities and experiences surfaced that, heretofore, would have remained hidden to visitors. One example occurred when the visitors asked faculty to describe activities that emphasized creativity and critical thinking. As part of a community health course, faculty negotiated with the owners of a chicken farm for students to orchestrate a health fair for its large number of employees. Students, working in groups, planned, implemented, and publicized the fair, and arranged for employee follow-up. Students and faculty learned a lot about the subculture of the chicken farm and about rural southern folkways; for example, the "old" hands held themselves separate from the "younger" workers even physically separating the working areas. Due to the subsequent media coverage, the program was besieged with requests from other industries. Students were able to participate in a reality-based situation, for which they were totally responsible and for which they used creative problem-solving and critical thinking. Under the previous rules and visitor routines, this learning activity would never have been brought to the attention of the visitors because it was not described in the written materials.

During another site visit, a neophyte faculty member wandered into the room in which site visitors were reviewing program materials. She wanted to discuss her course in pediatric nursing. She had arranged her classes according to the textbook, which was organized so that respiratory problems were covered at the end of the book. The course was offered in the winter quarter, with clinical practice held in a 1,000-bed teaching hospital. Following the textbook outline, as she thought she had to, would have put students in the problematic position of caring for a number of children with respiratory problems, all during the winter quarter, and connecting this with the classroom learning activities near the end of the quarter. She discussed how to organize her course better with the visitors. Such a shift in the use of visitor time seldom occurred under the old format.

Visitors also met with students and followed a similar format to the one used during the faculty meeting. It was interesting that students and faculty, independently, often mirrored each others comments about which learning activities were most meaningful. In some programs, however, learning activities occurred as a presorted package because "that was the way they were always done." In instances such as these, students risked falling into the trap of doing what was required to pass, not making waves, and graduating from a program in which training, not education had occurred. On more than one occasion, site visitors asked students to describe their most exciting learning activities and the result was dead silence. For the most part, however, silence has not occurred, and the meetings with students have become exciting parts of the site visits.

Site visits to clinical agencies have also changed as a result of the modification of the rules. Georgia nursing programs affiliate with over 500 agencies. In a 1987 rule revision, the Board ceased its approval, per se, of clinical agencies. Another state agency, analogous to the Board, has that responsibility. The Board has retained its authority to verify written descriptions of agencies used by a program. Site visits to agencies generally involved a meeting with the registered nurse responsible for nursing services and a breathless, hurried visit to several nursing units. The visitor would leave with an architectural sense of the agency and little else. During the 1990–1991 visits, the visitor met with the nursing administrator to discuss general characteristics of the agency and nursing service related to learning opportunities. Following this, a meeting was held with nursing representatives from the clinical units. These nurses were asked to describe their patient/client populations and to share clinical learning activities available on their units. Spirited and enthusiastic discussions resulted. A sleeper question concerning available legal, ethical, cultural, socioeconomic, and environmental safety learning activities produced a wealth of information. Tours of the agency were not done.

A tangential benefit of the new mode of agency site visits occurred in a city in which a new program was being developed. The education consultant suggested that faculty and agency staff brainstorm together about course development and clinical learning activities. The consultant was invited to attend the session, which was not only stimulating, but yielded collaborative commitment to classroom and clinical learning activities.

CONCLUSIONS

What has unfolded as a result of the rule changes is an increase in the already strong sense in Georgia that the Board of Nursing and its staff are allies with educators in the interest of quality education. They are seen less often as adversaries or policemen.

The Georgia Board of Nursing, its education consultant, and the Education Committee set out to test the water for dragons, to explore the spaces off the map in order to determine if regulation had to prescribe the behaviorist paradigm to be effective. It is becoming increasingly apparent that regulation can occur without strangulation. Freedom from some of the more prescriptive regulatory restraints need not mean that quality is sacrificed nor that education will lose the progress it has won with so much difficulty. If there is a boiling ocean, sea monsters, and dragons, they have not been encountered. Instead, a route is being explored to a regulatory environment conducive to creativity, critical thinking, and collaboration. The curriculum revolution and its accompanying emancipation of faculty and students and its emphasis on caring, creativity, and critical thinking can be used in programs without jeopardy to quality. Hugging the shore may seem safe, but routes to educational riches are incredibly productive.

REFERENCES

Bevis, E. (1973). *Curriculum building in nursing: A process*. St. Louis: C. V. Mosby.

Bevis, E. (1989). *Curriculum building in nursing: A process.* New York: National League for Nursing.

Bevis, E. & Watson, J. (1989). *Toward a caring curriculum: A new pedagogy for nursing.* New York: National League for Nursing.

Benner, P. (1984). *From novice to expert: Excellence and power in clinical nursing practice.* Menlo Park, Ca: Addison-Wesley Publishing Co.

Georgia Board of Nursing, (1987, 1989 & 1991). *Rules and regulations.* Atlanta: Georgia Board of Nursing.

Georgia Board of Nursing, (1990). *Georgia registered professional nurse practice act.* Atlanta: Georgia Board of Nursing.

Mager, R. (1962). *Preparing instructional objectives.* Belmont, CA: Feron Publishers.

Murray, J. (1989). *Developing criteria to support new curriculum models in nursing.* Unpublished doctoral dissertation, University of Georgia.

Sand, O. (1955). *Curriculum study in basic nursing education.* New York: G. P. Putnam's Sons.

Tyler, R. (1949). *Basic principles of curriculum and instruction.* Chicago: University of Chicago Press.